# More Advance Praise for
## *Neurocritical Care*

W9-BHV-321

"The essence of the contemporary clinical practice of Critical Care Neurology is rapidly making life-and-death decisions for patients with conditions about which there is often little conclusive clinical science available for guidance. In this unique text, Drs. Wijdicks and Rabinstein—true masters of both the practice and science of critical care neurology—deftly combine nuanced interpretation of the most pertinent scientific literature with unparalleled experience and incisive reasoning to provide explicit guidance for making the most difficult of these decisions. *Neurocritical Care* is written in a style that makes it suitable for both reading in its entirety and as a reference. It is a must-read for anyone who regularly cares for critically ill neurologic and neurosurgical patients. Furthermore, due to its pragmatic approach, it should be readily available in all emergency departments and intensive care units as a first-line reference when a difficult neurocritical care issue arises."

> —*Joseph D. Burns, MD, Attending Neurointensivist, Boston Medical Center, Department of Neurology and Neurosurgery, Boston University School of Medicine*

"*Neurocritical Care* by Wijdicks and Rabinstein is an innovative and highly effective text to educate physicians about this rapidly growing field. The book is original and practical; it approaches the educational matter in a real-life manner, with the presentation of cases followed by honest and down-to-earth discussions of the basics and nuances of management. The book reminds me of another authoritative text: Adams, Victor, and Ropper's *Neurology*, also admirable for its readability and practical advice. Wijdicks and Rabinstein provide the appropriate amount of evidence for the reader to understand the essentials of management, but without going into so much detail as to bore or confuse the reader. They provide "key points" at the culmination of each chapter, giving the reader salient take-home messages that allow for easy digestion. They also provide recommendations for further reading on given subjects, often pointing to the sentinel articles on a subject, or to excellent review articles that will assist the reader as they attempt to expand their knowledge base. In an age in which it is difficult to know what to read that is authoritative and yet not overly exhaustive or time-consuming, *Neurocritical Care* is refreshingly straightforward and downright enjoyable to read. It should be a staple on every neurologist's or critical care physician's desk."

> —*David M. Greer, MD, MA, FCCM, Vice Chair, Department of Neurology, Yale University School of Medicine*

# What Do I Do Now?

SERIES CO-EDITORS-IN-CHIEF

**Lawrence C. Newman, MD**
Director of the Headache Institute
Department of Neurology
St. Luke's-Roosevelt Hospital Center
New York, NY

**Morris Levin, MD**
Co-director of the Dartmouth Headache Center
Director of the Dartmouth Neurology Residency Training Program
Section of Neurology
Dartmouth Hitchcock Medical Center
Lebanon, NH

PREVIOUS VOLUMES IN THE SERIES

*Headache and Facial Pain*
*Peripheral Nerve and Muscle Disease*
*Pediatric Neurology*
*Stroke*
*Epilepsy*

# Neurocritical Care

**Eelco F. M. Wijdicks, MD, PhD, FACP**
Professor of Neurology, College of Medicine
Chair, Division of Critical Care Neurology
Consultant, Neurosciences Intensive Care Unit
Saint Marys Hospital, Mayo Clinic
Rochester, Minnesota

**Alejandro A. Rabinstein, MD**
Professor of Neurology, College of Medicine
Division of Critical Care Neurology
Medical Director and Consultant
Neurosciences Intensive Care Unit
Saint Marys Hospital, Mayo Clinic
Rochester, Minnesota

OXFORD
UNIVERSITY PRESS

# OXFORD
UNIVERSITY PRESS

Oxford University Press, Inc., publishes works that further Oxford University's objective of excellence
in research, scholarship, and education.

Oxford   New York
Auckland   Cape Town   Dar es Salaam   Hong Kong   Karachi   Kuala Lumpur   Madrid
Melbourne   Mexico City   Nairobi   New Delhi   Shanghai   Taipei   Toronto

With offices in
Argentina   Austria   Brazil   Chile   Czech Republic   France   Greece   Guatemala   Hungary   Italy
Japan   Poland   Portugal   Singapore   South Korea   Switzerland   Thailand   Turkey   Ukraine   Vietnam

Copyright © 2012 by Mayo Foundation for Medical Education and Research

Published by Oxford University Press, Inc.
198 Madison Avenue, New York, New York 10016
www.oup.com

First issued as an Oxford University Press paperback, 2012

Oxford is a registered trademark of Oxford University Press

Library of Congress Cataloging-in-Publication Data

Wijdicks, Eelco F. M., 1954-
Neurocritical care / Eelco F. M. Wijdicks, Alejandro A. Rabinstein.
    p. ; cm. — (What do I do now?)
Includes bibliographical references.
ISBN 978-0-19-984362-6 (pbk)   1.  Neurological intensive care.   I.  Rabinstein, Alejandro A.   II.  Title.
III.  Series: What do I do now?
[DNLM: 1.  Nervous System Diseases—therapy.   2.  Critical Care--methods.
3.  Emergency Medicine. 4.  Intensive Care Units. 5.  Trauma, Nervous System—therapy.  WL 140]
RC350.N49W5497 2012
616.8'0428—dc23                     2011014390

The science of medicine is a rapidly changing field. As new research and clinical experience broaden our
knowledge, changes in treatment and drug therapy occur. The author and publisher of this work have checked
with sources believed to be reliable in their efforts to provide information that is accurate and complete, and
in accordance with the standards accepted at the time of publication. However, in light of the possibility of
human error or changes in the practice of medicine, neither the author, nor the publisher, nor any other party
who has been involved in the preparation or publication of this work warrants that the information contained
herein is in every respect accurate or complete. Readers are encouraged to confirm the information contained
herein with other reliable sources, and are strongly advised to check the product information sheet provided
by the pharmaceutical company for each drug they plan to administer.

9 8 7 6 5 4 3 2 1

Printed in the United States of America on acid-free paper

To our beautiful wives Barbara and Carlota

To the delightful nursing staff of the Neurosciences Intensive Care Unit
—EFMW and AAR

And to the memory of my mother. She defined who I am.
—AAR

# Preface

Critical care neurology (*NEUROCRITICAL CARE*) is an established subspecialty, and the field relates to treating patients with an acute and serious neurologic illness. This broad discipline involves many well-defined neurologic disorders and their medical complications, and the practice is somewhere in between *NEURO*critical care and neuro*CRITICAL CARE*. All patients need close observation and management of emerging problems, some need a neurosurgical intervention or a neurointerventional procedure, a few patients are in extremis, but all need comprehensive care in a—preferably—neurosciences intensive care unit (NICU).

Neurointensivists are busy deciders. Attending in the NICU is filled with answering calls, acute interventions, and making informed decisions impacting direction of care. Problems can rather quickly spin out of control and it is therefore quite fitting to have *NEUROCRITICAL CARE* represented in this series on what to do next when the presenting problem is not a simple matter.

We have approached this handbook differently than the prior books we wrote and edited. First, we tried not to run the risk of repeating all the issues one more time and we wanted to say something new about common critical neurologic problems. Second, we have tried to stay evidence-based wherever we can. Third, from the initial treatment of serious neurologic disorders to end-of-life care discussions, this book addresses mostly interventions. All medical complications are specifically related to neurologic patients, and the cases may help any physician to tackle these problems head-on before asking for help. The case descriptions here are about patients we cared for in the NICU and about patients in other intensive care units when we were consulted for advice on diagnosis and management.

We wrote it as if we were at morning rounds, at the bedside to make a decision or on the phone discussing changes in care and setting goals. Each case ends with additional information, and this book provides over 100 reputable references that should be in every physician's PDF library.

Our experience is thoroughly steeped in a neurology education, and this book is therefore expectedly directed toward neurologists, neurosurgeons, residents, and fellows. And, yet residents of all specialties or residents just starting off and rotating through the NICU should anticipate these problems and they may want a quick educational read before they jump in. Seasoned physicians may find some relevant material here, too.

This collection of cases tries to give the right weight to the complexity of care and new approaches of management. It is obvious that this concise book is not a substitute for anything, and other comprehensive works should be consulted. We can only scratch the surface here and make a few points. We have tried to fill the pages with practical suggestions for each topic it covers and hope this handbook can be used for teaching case examples. Ultimately it may ignite interest in the field. So start reading, immerse yourself, and see what you think.

E.F.M. Wijdicks
A.A. Rabinstein

# Contents

## SECTION II CALLS, PAGES, AND OTHER ALARMS

## SECTION III LONG-TERM SUPPORT, END-OF-LIFE CARE, AND PALLIATION

# Neurocritical Care

# Acute Interventions

# 1  Surgery for Cerebral Hemorrhage

A 56-year-old man with history of hypertension presented to our emergency department with complaints of severe headache and visual changes. At the first encounter his level of alertness was normal and his only neurological deficit was a right visual field deficit. His blood pressure was 194/112 mmHg. He was treated with intravenous labetalol. Shortly after his arrival he became sleepier, and repeat examination showed right-sided weakness and hypoesthesia. An emergency CT scan showed a large left lobar hematoma (estimated volume 65 cm$^3$) with regional mass effect. (Figure 1.1A) Coagulation values were normal. The blood pressure remained elevated despite repeated doses of labetalol, but became finally better controlled after initiation of a nicardipine infusion.

When we see the patient in the emergency department immediately after the CT scan he is arousable to strong voice but does not remain awake unless he is stimulated. His pupils are symmetric and reactive to light. He does not blink to visual threat on the right and has a moderate right hemiparesis and sensory loss. He has a right Babinski sign, but plantar response remains flexor on the left.

**What do you do now?**

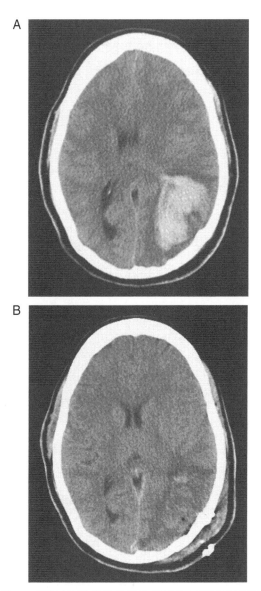

**FIGURE 1.1** A) CT scan of the head before surgical evacuation showing a large left lobar hematoma with extensive regional mass effect. B) Complete evacuation of the hematoma with resolution of the mass effect is shown in a CT scan obtained 72 hours after surgery.

No doubt this is a disconcerting clinical situation. Most of us know that surgery for cerebral hematoma—dissecting through healthy neuronal tissue to reach the clot—is no sinecure. There is evidence that surgery does not improve outcome in deep seated ganglionic hemorrhages but faced with a patient worsening from a lobar hematoma a more nuanced understanding is necessary. Here is some useful information to help in making a decision.

Intracerebral hemorrhage (ICH) often has devastating consequences. Four in ten patients with ICH die, and many survivors can remain disabled. Furthermore, the medical treatment of ICH is limited to supportive care, control of severe hypertension, and correction of coagulation abnormalities when present. In patients with spontaneous ICH, hemostatic therapy reduces hematoma expansion, but has not been proven to result in better functional outcomes. Some hematoma enlargements do not translate in measurable clinical differences, or the treatment—mostly recombinant factor VIIa—may be helpful only in patients who continue to bleed. The challenge now for clinical researchers is to identify patients who would benefit most. Therefore, the combination of poor prognosis and lack of effective medical therapy makes the alternative of a surgical intervention appealing. Yet, multiple studies comparing medical and surgical management of spontaneous ICH have shown disappointing results.

The largest trial evaluating surgical evacuation for spontaneous ICH was the Surgical Trial in Intracerebral Hemorrhage (STICH). Over 500 patients—with similar numbers of hematomas in the putamen/thalamus and lobar locations—were randomized to surgical or medical treatment within 3 days of ICH onset (median time to surgery was 30 hours). Six months later, only one quarter of patients in both groups had achieved good recovery or had no more than moderate disability. Therefore, surgery did not improve the outcome of patients with spontaneous ICH at large, which confirmed the results of previous smaller trials. Subgroup analyses in the STICH population however, disclosed that patients who were not comatose and had superficial lobar hematomas (< 1 cm from the brain surface) did better when they underwent surgery. Patients with these characteristics are currently being enrolled in another trial (STICH II).

We need to keep in mind that trials evaluating surgery in ICH have typically not enrolled rapidly deteriorating patients (in fact, "rescue" surgery took place in more than one in four patients randomized to the medical group in the STICH trial). Although in three quarters of patients outcome is still poor, we have seen patients with signs of clinical and radiological brainstem compression or displacement who recovered well after emergency evacuation. If those patients have good potential for recovery, surgery should at least be considered.

We know a few other things about surgery for ICH. Deep-seated hematomas do not benefit from evacuation via a traditional open craniotomy but some case series and one randomized study indicated that stereotactic surgery with needle aspiration could be useful in deep seated hematoma. The safety and efficacy of stereotactic evacuation facilitated by instillation of a thrombolytic agent into the hematoma to liquefy it requires further evaluation of experience in this regard is limited. Ultra-early hematoma evacuation was a concept that made a lot of sense a priori, but a clinical trial testing this strategy had to be terminated because of increased numbers of deaths among patients operated within hours. This was explained by difficulty to maintain hemostasis and frequent postoperative rebleeding. On the other hand, hovering between "wait and see" or "do something" to then proceed with a surgical intervention only after the patient has become comatose from mass effect seems poor practice. Surgery was ineffective in comatose patients in STICH. Furthermore, in reality, waiting for the patient to decline before offering surgery often results in not offering surgery at all. Once the patient is "too poor for surgery" the opportunity is gone.

Surgery is standard practice in certain circumstances. We do know that sizable cerebellar hematomas must be evacuated to avoid obstructive hydrocephalus and brainstem compression, all of which can be fatal or result in irreversible complications. Delaying evacuation of the clot in these patients is ill-advised.

Another population in which surgery is indicated is when the ICH is secondary to a vascular anomaly (such as an arteriovenous malformation or an aneurysm) because of the high risk of recurrent bleeding, and when there is suspicion of an underlying tumor. Generally, suspicion of amyloid angiopathy does not contraindicate surgery (in the past the fragility of the arteries has worried neurosurgeons). Some patients with pathologically confirmed amyloid angiopathy can recover well after surgery, especially those younger than 75 years, without intraventricular hemorrhage, and without history of dementia.

Another neurosurgical issue is the placement of a ventriculostomy in a patient with cerebral hematoma and obstructive hydrocephalus. This intervention seldom results in clinical improvement because obstructive hydrocephalus is often the result of a large clot compressing the ventricles. CSF diversion alone in these cases is not sufficient.

So what did we decide to do with our patient? Neurosurgery was consulted in the emergency department. We discussed the situation with the family, since the patient was not able to sustain attention sufficiently to participate in the conversation we told them that we had a favorable experience with early intervention, but without scientific proof of benefit. We mentioned that later surgery would not be a good option. After the family provided informed consent, our neurosurgical team performed a craniotomy and clot evacuation. Surgery started 6 hours after patient presentation and approximately 8 hours after symptom onset and achieved successful hematoma evacuation. The following day the patient was awake and could be safely extubated. He was discharged from the hospital with a right visual deficit and minimal right arm weakness and numbness. He continued to improve and was back to work 6 months later, and this time he was taking his antihypertensive medications (unlike before the ICH, when he had been noncompliant).

When considering surgery for ICH, we need to take into account various factors related to the ICH itself, the patient's chances of recovery, and the patient's preferences, which often have to be discussed with the family or proxy (Table 1.1). When the decision is to go to surgery, first the patient needs to be fully stabilized (i.e., adequate ventilation and oxygenation, control of hypertension below a systolic blood pressure of 180–160 mmHg, and correction of anticoagulation as discussed in chapter 2). Realistic expectations are discussed with the family. In many cases, surgery may reduce mortality but without improving function. While some cases can get better when the clot is removed, as illustrated by our example, in most situations surgery is far from a standard approach for these patients. Careful patient selection is probably the key to optimizing functional results, but we still do not know which patients are the best candidates for surgical treatment. Yet, if surgery is being considered, one should not wait until the patient markedly worsens.

**TABLE 1.1** Factors Favoring Surgery for ICH

Worsening clinical signs

Young age

Absence of severe comorbidities

Absent or corrected coagulopathy

Lobar hematoma
  (< 1 cm from brain surface)

Absent brainstem injury

Absent intraventricular hemorrhage

Good rehabilitation potential

---

**KEY POINTS TO REMEMBER REGARDING SURGERY FOR CEREBRAL HEMORRHAGE**

- Surgery cannot be recommended as a routine intervention for patients with spontaneous ICH.
- Selected patients with spontaneous ICH might benefit from surgery, especially noncomatose patients with good rehabilitation potential and superficial hematomas without associated intraventricular hemorrhage.
- When surgery is considered, it is most reasonable to perform it early, but in stable patients preferably not during the first 4 hours after ICH onset because of problems with hemostasis in this ultra-early period.
- Surgery is indicated in patients with large cerebellar hematomas, and underlying vascular anomalies or tumors.

**Further Reading**

Mendelow AD, Gregson BA, Fernandes HM, Murray GD, Teasdale GM, Hope DT, Karimi A, Shaw MD, Barer DH, STICH investigators. Early surgery versus initial conservative treatment in patients with spontaneous supratentorial intracerebral hematomas in the International Surgical Trial in Intracerebral Hemorrhage (STICH): a randomized trial. *Lancet* 2005; 365:387-397.

Petridis AK, Barth H, Buhl R, Hugo HH, Mehdorn HM. Outcome of cerebral amyloid angiopathic brain hemorrhage. *Acta Neurochir (Wien)* 2008; 150:889-895.

Prasad K, Mendelow AD, Gregson B. Surgery for primary supratentorial intracerebral hemorrhage. *Cochrane Database Syst Rev* 2008; 8(4):CD000200.

Rabinstein AA, Atkinson JL, Wijdicks EFM. Emergency craniotomy in patients worsening due to expanded cerebral hematoma: to what purpose? *Neurology* 2002; 58: 1367-1372.

Rabinstein AA, Wijdicks EFM. Surgery for intracerebral hematoma: the search for the elusive right candidate. *Rev Neurol Dis* 2006; 3:163-172.

Rabinstein AA, Wijdicks EFM. Determinants of outcome in anticoagulation-associated cerebral hematoma requiring emergency evacuation. *Arch Neurol* 2007; 64: 203-206.

# Reversal of Anticoagulation After Cerebral Hemorrhage

A 70-year-old man with a metallic aortic valve treated with warfarin and aspirin developed a sudden speech difficulty, right-arm weakness and numbness. On arrival to an outside emergency department he was alert, but there was a severe dysarthria and right-sided hemiparesis involving arm and leg. CT scan showed a localized thalamic hematoma without ventricular extension, but with some mass effect (Figure 2.1). International normalized ratio (INR) was 4.3. He received fresh frozen plasma (2 units) and intravenous vitamin K (5 mg). The neurosurgeon at the outside hospital felt there was no surgical option and would only intervene after INR was corrected.

After transfer to our emergency department, there was clear evidence of further neurologic deterioration, mainly decline in responsiveness with eye opening to voice only, impaired vertical eye movements, marked dysarthria, and flaccid hemiparesis. He is still able to protect his airway, but he has developed Cheyne-Stokes breathing. Repeat CT scan of the brain shows enlargement of the thalamic hematoma and rupture into the third ventricle. His systolic blood pressure has climbed to 200 mmHg. INR is still 4.0.

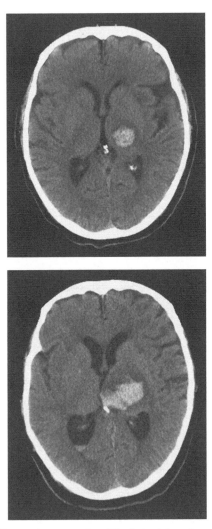

**FIGURE 2.1** Serial CT scans show expansion of the thalamic hematoma and development of acute hydrocephalus.

Ongoing anticoagulation in a patient with a cerebral hematoma is a serious concern. As expected, warfarin causes larger cerebral hemorrhages and increases the chance of poor outcome. Avoiding this expansion—and even reduction of size by 2 teaspoons could make a difference—may reduce the morbidity from additional brain tissue destruction or prevent brainstem injury from displacement. Everyone would agree that a first step would be to quickly correct the INR to a normal value (INR < 1.5). However, it is not well established that rapid reversal of the anticoagulant effects of warfarin effectively reduces enlargement of the hematoma.

The approach is to reverse the antagonistic effect of warfarin on vitamin K, and vitamin K will then reactivate factors II, VII, IX, and X. Using both intravenous vitamin K and fresh frozen plasma (FFP) accomplishes that, but only after several hours. Moreover, vitamin K alone is not sufficient and may even take 6–24 hours to take full effect; therefore by itself vitamin K has no substantial effect on expansion of the hematoma occurring usually in the first hours after the initial hemorrhage. FFP further replaces the depleted coagulation factors, but multiple studies have shown that target INR is not reached within 2–4 hours in the majority of patients (compatibility testing and thawing of plasma lasting 30–60 minutes adds to the delay). Equally problematic is when INR is not corrected rapidly with FFP, since it may lead physicians to infuse more units of FFP, since leading to transfusion-associated circulatory overload, pulmonary edema, and in the worst-case scenario endotracheal intubation and mechanical ventilation. There is no consensus on the number of FFP units needed, although weight-based calculation may reduce complications. As a general rule, a dose of 10–20 mL of FFP/kg of body weight will produce a sufficient 10% increase in coagulation factors. A typical unit is 250 cc, thus 3 to 4 units are often needed. Finally and most concerning, one should not be surprised to find out that some emergency departments may not have fresh frozen plasma readily available. This delay in treatment is obviously unacceptable.

The best alternative options for correction of warfarin are prothrombin complex concentrate (PCC) or recombinant activated factor VII (rFVIIa). PCCs contain human derived clotting factors and rFVIIa is bioengineered. PCCs are basically a concentrate of factor IX and smaller amounts of II, X, and VII. Neither PCC nor rFVIIa is universally available.

There is a tendency to prefer PCC (Table 2.1). There are several reasons for that: it is easy to use and quickly prepared, there is a minimal infused volume, it nearly completely replaces clotting factors, and the most convincing argument for some physicians is that it lasts longer than rFVIIa and less additional FFP may be needed. But thrombotic events using PCC may not be different from rFVIIa, and there are very few studies that have assessed this risk with PCC. The risk of arterial and venous occlusive events in rFVIIa was 26% with a low dose (20 mcg/kg) and almost 50% with higher dose (80 mcg/kg) in the largest cerebral hematoma trial although most of these events were inconsequential. This is consistent with our experience in daily practice. A recent detailed analysis of several clinical trials in multiple conditions found these increased risks, particularly in patients over 65 years of age, often resulting in venous occlusions.

Patients with severe thrombocytopenia need platelet transfusions. An unresolved issue is whether platelet infusion in a patient with prior use of antiplatelet agents reduces hematoma expansion or improves outcome. Clinical trials are underway, and there is yet no definite evidence that platelet infusion can impact on progression of the hemorrhage or even outcome.

A new problem will be introduced when the use of dabigatran (a thrombin or factor II inhibitor) or apixaban (a factor Xa inhibitor) becomes more commonplace, because no reversal strategy is available other than stopping

TABLE 2.1  **Reversal of Warfarin**

|  | IV Vit K | FFP | PCC | rFVIIa |
|---|---|---|---|---|
| Dose | 5-10 mg | 10-40 mL/kg | 25-50 U/kg | 20-40 mcg/kg* |
| INR Correction | delayed | rapid | rapid | rapid |
| Disadvantage | none | large volume/ thawing time | thrombogenic | thrombogenic |
| Preference | † | † | †† | † |

† = commonly used
†† = preferred, if available, there may be substantial differences in costs between products
* Much lower doses (5-10 mcg/kg) may be sufficient in our experience

the drug. The anticoagulation effect of these newer drugs reverses many hours (half life 12–15 hours) after discontinuation and thus not soon enough. FFP would not have any major effect, but PCC or rFVIIa may help. Research on antibodies against these drugs is ongoing. Finding an antidote will be important because these new expensive drugs may replace warfarin in the long run.

So what should you do? Table 2.2 summarizes the initial priorities. The initial management must remain focused on rapid correction of the INR. Equally important is aggressive control of blood pressure using labetalol, hydralazine, or intravenous infusion with nicardipine with the assumption that keeping the blood pressure under control additionally reduces further expansion.

Another potential complication in patients with a thalamic hemorrhage is the development of hydrocephalus due to trapping of CSF outflow at the foramen of Monro. A ventriculostomy is readily placed by neurosurgeons— after INR correction—in patients with significant intraventricular clot, but there is serious doubt if this intervention can change outcome or even result in a noticeable improvement. (In some patients the diencephalic destruction may leave the patient in a prolonged stuporous state and a ventriculostomy does not help.) Acute hydrocephalus may be a reflection of a major hemorrhage and not necessarily a treatable complication. Moreover, keeping the ventriculostomy patent and draining has always been the limiting factor. In patients with a lobar hematoma and worsening neurological findings, surgical evacuation is the only available option for survival.

**TABLE 2.2  Emergency Management of Warfarin Associated Cerebral Hemorrhage**

Aggressively lower INR to normal (INR < 1.5)

Aggressively control blood pressure (SBP < 160 mmHg)

Consider ventriculostomy when INR < 1.5 and hemoventricle with hydrocephalus

Monitor EKG/troponin if rFVIIa has been administered

Monitor X-Ray of the chest for pulmonary infiltrates if FFP has been used and consider diuretics

Outcome therefore will be determined by 1) whether the appropriate interventions are pursued in a salvageable patient and 2) sufficient time for recovery is allowed.

But what of resumption of anticoagulation after the patient recovers and still needs protection against future emboli? The risk of future hemorrhagic complications after resuming warfarin is 10–20%. Early thromboembolic complications have been estimated at 5%. There is no clear consensus on what to do and the trade-off depends on the individual risk of thromboembolism (higher with prosthetic valves) and recurrent hemorrhage (higher with suspected cerebral amyloid angiopathy). One retrospective analysis—mostly in patients with atrial fibrillation alone—found that waiting 1–2 months was justified. Others have found that even waiting with restarting anticoagulation for 7–10 days has resulted in increase in thrombotic complications and have recommended that one should consider restarting low intensity warfarin 3–4 days after the patient has a stable hematoma and no neurosurgical intervention has been performed. While taking the risk of restarting warfarin so promptly may be unnecessary in most cases, early resumption of warfarin may be considered in patients with prior TIAs, prosthetic valves, or echocardiographic finding of an atrial thrombus. We generally wait 7–10 days before restarting.

---

**KEY POINTS TO REMEMBER REGARDING WARFARIN ASSOCIATED CEREBRAL HEMORRHAGES**

- PCC or rFVIIa may be a more effective way to reverse warfarin.
- Vitamin K and fresh frozen plasma may be the only available option, but INR is corrected in only 1/3 of the patients within 12 hours.
- Control of blood pressure is equally important to reduce expansion of the hematoma.
- Ventriculostomy may be needed in patients with significant intraventricular blood, but only when INR is less than 1.5.
- Neurosurgical evacuation of hematoma should remain an option, but only when INR is less than 1.5.

## Further Reading

Aguilar MI, Hart RG, Kase CS, Freeman WD et al. Treatment of warfarin-associated intracerebral hemorrhage: literature review of expert opinion. *Mayo Clin Proc* 2007; 82:82-92.

Bershad EM, Suarez JI. Prothrombin complex concentrates for oral anticoagulant therapy-related intracranial hemorrhage: a review of the literature. *Neurocrit Care* 2010; 12:403-413.

Claassen DO, Kazemi N, Zubkov AY, Wijdicks EFM, Rabinstein AA. Restarting anticoagulation therapy after warfarin-associated intracerebral hemorrhage. *Arch Neurol* 2008; 65:1313-1318.

Diringer MN, Skolnick BE, Mayer SA, Steiner T, Davis SM, Brun NC, Broderick JP. Thromboembolic events with recombinant activated factor VII in spontaneous intracerebral hemorrhage: results from the Factor Seven for Acute Hemorrhagic Stroke (FAST) trial. *Stroke* 2010; 41:48-53.

Elliott J, Smith M. The acute management of intracerebral hemorrhage: a clinical review. *Anesth Analg* 2010; 110:1419-1427.

Imberti D, Barillari G, Baisoli C et al. Emergency reversal of anticoagulation with a three-factor prothrombin complex concentrate in patients with intracranial hemorrhage. *Blood Transfus* 2011;9:148-155.

Lee SB, Manno EM, Layton KF, Wijdicks EFM. Progression of warfarin-associated intracerebral hemorrhage after INR normalization with FFP. *Neurology* 2006; 67:1272-1274.

Levi M, Levy JH, Andersen HF, Truloff VM. Safety of recombinant activated factor VII in randomized clinical trials. *N Engl J Med* 2010; 363:1791-1800.

Majeed A, Kim Y-K, Roberts RS. Optimal timing of resumption of warfarin after intracranial hemorrhage. *Stroke* 2010; 41:2860-2866.

Robinson MT, Rabinstein AA, Meschia JF et al. Safety of recombinant activated factor VII in patients with warfarin-associated hemorrhages of the central nervous system. *Stroke* 2010; 41:1459-1463.

Steiner T, Bosel J. Options to restrict hematoma expansion after spontaneous intracerebral hemorrhage. *Stroke* 2010; 41:402-409.

# 3 Medical Care of Traumatic Brain Injury

A 22-year-old patient was in a bar fight and got hit in the head multiple times. He was intubated by a paramedic. On arrival, he is comatose. There are marked bruises in his face and swollen eyelids. His eyes are not opening to pain. Pupils are small, but with good light responses. Corneal reflexes cannot not be obtained, and oculocephalic reflexes cannot not be tested due to uncertainty of associated spine injury. The other brainstem reflexes are intact. There is extensor posturing. CT scan shows evidence of multiple contusions in the frontal and temporal lobes. There is no evidence of a subdural or epidural hematoma. CT of the cervical spine is normal. His alcohol level is markedly increased at 0.3%. Initial examination does not reveal any other systemic injury or fractures, and his vital signs are stable. Arterial blood gas is normal.

*What do you do now?*

I t is of primary importance to understand the causes and consequences of coma in a patient with a traumatic brain injury. Think—at least—of five crucial issues.

*First issue*: One has to determine whether neurosurgical intervention is needed. Urgent neurosurgical indications are often obvious at the time of arrival and usually involve the presence of a large cerebral contusion creating mass effect and brain tissue displacement. The presence of an acute subdural or epidural hematoma on admission CT scan is always neurosurgical terrain (Figure 3.1). Be warned, these hematomas can emerge quickly, and a normal CT scan after any significant trauma may not mean much. A repeat CT scan should be performed if the clinical examination does not fit the neuroimaging findings, and perhaps the threshold should be even lower in intoxicated patients. A depressed skull fracture will need to be explored by the neurosurgeon.

*Second issue:* Is the patient actively bleeding? Some patients are on warfarin and this will need to be reversed immediately with vitamin K, and, because of the urgency and possible surgery, with recombinant activated factor VII or prothrombin complex concentrate. Most neurosurgeons prefer an INR of less than 1.5 before surgery.

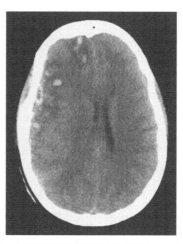

**FIGURE 3.1** Early CT scan after traumatic brain injury showing major contusional lesions and subdural hematomas with mass effect.

*Third issue:* There are often major confounders—as it is alcohol intoxication in our case example. A toxicology screen may be needed but a careful history remains most valuable. It is unlikely that the current presentation of extensor posturing is explained by alcohol, but his level of responsiveness could be markedly confounded with such ethanol level in the blood. (This level is lethal in a naive drinker and therefore indicates that the patient is a chronic alcoholic.)

*Fourth issue:* Any comatose patient after traumatic brain injury (TBI) is at high risk of increased intracranial pressure. Options are an intraparenchymal probe or a ventriculostomy. Most major trauma centers use a fiberoptic device that measures ICP. A ventriculostomy can be placed, but in patients with a small ventricle size and risk of further compression, this is a second target of approach. Placement of an intraparenchymal ICP monitor provides not only an intracranial pressure value, but also the cerebral perfusion pressure (CPP) that can be calculated knowing the mean arterial blood pressure (MAP). The abbreviated formula is CCP = MAP - ICP. The optimal ICP and CPP are currently defined as an ICP less than 20 mmHg and a CPP between 50 and 70 mmHg.

Indications for intracranial monitoring have been well set and include patients with a severe TBI defined as coma, decerebrate, or decorticate posturing, and an abnormal CT scan (contusions, shear lesions, early brain edema). Any patient that will require deep sedation—usually when pulmonary injury is present—is probably best managed by monitoring intracranial pressure. The value of brain tissue oxygen monitoring using an additional intraparenchymal probe to guide the management of TBI has not been established.

*Fifth issue:* Treatment of increased intracranial pressure first requires mundane interventions such as aggressive oxygenation, avoidance of hypercarbia, treatment of posttraumatic seizures, but also reducing intrathoracic (PEEP values less than 15 mmHg) and intra-abdominal pressure. Fentanyl 1 mg/kg per hour, atracurium 0.5 mg/kg per hour or midazolam 0.1 mg/kg per hour might be necessary to adequately sedate the patient and have the patient synchronize the mechanical ventilator. Although commonly used in TBI, the effect of opiates on ICP is variable, and we have seen patients with reduced intracranial compliance in which the ICP increased after the administration of these drugs. Seizures will have to be treated, and baseline

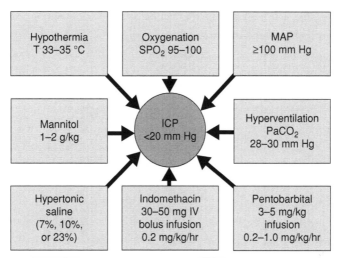

**FIGURE 3.2** Optimizing conditions and treatment for increased intracranial pressure (modified from Wijdicks, *The Comatose Patient*. Oxford University Press, New York, 2008).

EEG might be necessary if focal seizures have occurred. It is common practice to treat more severely injured stuporous or comatose patient with IV levetiracetam or, less preferably, fosphenytoin (Figure 3.2).

Treatment of intracranial pressure is best first managed with hyperventilation (arterial PCO2 in the 30s) and mannitol using 1 to 2 g/kg. The use of hypertonic saline requires the placement of a central venous catheter, and waiting for that to be in place could markedly delay initial treatment of ICP. In equivalent osmolar doses, mannitol and hypertonic saline appear to have comparable effects on ICP and CPP. However, hypertonic saline can be administered in higher concentrations (23.4%), which can be effective even after mannitol or lower concentrations of hypertonic saline have failed to reduce ICP.

There is controversy whether hypothermia may improve outcome. Earlier studies showed better outcome after aggressive treatment with hypothermia, but this was not confirmed by subsequent larger clinical trials. The effect of hypothermia on ICP management, however, is substantial and has been repeatedly documented. Therefore, moderate hypothermia (33–35 degrees Celsius) is an eloquent way of reducing ICP as an additional treatment to the usual ICP-lowering agents.

Any unsuccessful control of ICP will have to be treated with decompressive craniectomy; either bifrontal craniectomy or hemicraniectomy. In extreme situations, patients with refractory ICP have benefited from abdominal decompression. The initial experience with decompressive craniectomy has shown significant reduction in ICP surges, but a recent randomized trial using bifrontotemporoparietal decompressive surgery found no improvement in outcome (the patient selection in this trial has been criticized because patients could be considered candidates for surgery after already 15 minutes of refractory ICP). Another trial (RESCUEicp) is ongoing.

A long-standing discussion has been whether treatment of traumatic head injury should be "ICP or CPP driven." Studies have not found any difference between these two approaches. However, treatment of CPP alone with less attention to increased intracranial pressure may be a wrong approach. It is not only cerebral perfusion that matters, and increasing ICP will eventually lead to brainstem displacement and permanent brainstem injury.

Treatment of TBI also involves other aspects of care (Table 3.1). Some have argued that in the most severe cases prophylactic placement of a

TABLE 3.1  **Initial Priorities after Traumatic Brain Injury**

*Need for ICP Control?*

Osmotic diuretics, Mannitol (20%, 1-2 g/kg) or Hypertonic Saline (30 ml of 23%)

Hyperventilation (short term and $PaCO_2$ around 30 mmHg)

Hypothermia (cooling device set to 33-34°C)

Decompressive surgery (Bifrontotemporoparietal craniectomy; evacuation of subdural hematoma or contusion with mass effect)

*Need for seizure control?*

Levetiracetam loading 2000 mg IV in cerebral contusions, increased ICP and skull fractures.

*Need for better oxygenation?*

Endotracheal intubation and mechanical ventilation

Careful use of PEEP

Midazolam infusion for sedation.

vena cava filter is a better option than waiting for pulmonary emboli to occur. In many of these patients, treatment with subcutaneous heparin may not suffice and may potentially increase the probability of hemorrhage in blossoming cerebral contusions. There is little consensus on how to proceed in such patients and how to identify those at very high risk of fatal pulmonary emboli. Filter placement may be an option if long-term care is anticipated in polytraumatized patients.

Gastrointestinal prophylaxis is essential for patients on a mechanical ventilator who have a substantial risk of gastrointestinal bleeding. Patients should be placed on lansoprazole or famotidine (a component of the "ventilator bundle").

Much of the treatment in TBI is recognition and early treatment of infections. This includes ventilator-associated pneumonia, urinary tract infections, but also catheter (line) sepsis; all complications that need to be treated appropriately. Early tracheostomy (and reducing time on the ventilator), close monitoring of intravascular catheters and prompt removal when infected or no longer necessary, surveillance for the development of deep venous thrombosis in upper and lower extremities, and early placement of a gastrostomy may all reduce complications and improve the chances of survival and functional outcome in general.

---

**KEY POINTS TO REMEMBER ABOUT TRAUMATIC BRAIN INJURY**

- Place an ICP monitor in any comatose patient with early CT scan abnormalities.
- Maintain ICP less than 20 mmHg and CPP between 60 and 70 mmHg (CPP is MAP - ICP).
- Hypertonic saline requires central access and has become a preferred method to quickly and effectively lower ICP.
- Last resort measures are induced hypothermia or decompressive craniectomy in refractory ICP
- Treat infections aggressively.
- Think early about other prophylactic measures (GI protection and surveillance for DVT).

## Further Reading

Brain Traumatic Foundation; American Association of Neurological Surgeons; Congress of Neurological Surgeons; Joint section on Neurotrauma and Critical Care, AANS/CNS, Bratton SL, Chestnut RM, Ghajar J, McConnell Hammond FF, Harris OA, Hartl R et al. Guidelines for the management of severe traumatic brain injury. VI. Indications for intracranial pressure monitoring. *J Neurotrauma* 2008; 24: S37-44.

Cooper DJ, Rosenfeld JV, Murray L, et al. Decompressive craniectomy in diffuse traumatic brain injury. *N Engl J Med*. 2011;364:1493-1502.

Dietrich WD, Bramlett HM. The evidence for hypothermia as a neuroprotectant in traumatic brain injury. *Neurotherapeutics* 2010; 7: 43-50.

Hijaz TA, Cento EA, Walker MT. Imaging of head trauma. *Radiol Clin North Am* 2010; 49:81-103.

Kamel H, Navi BB, Nakagawa K et al. Hypertonic saline versus mannitol for the treatment of elevated intracranial pressure: a meta-analysis of randomized clinical trials. Crit Care Med 2011;39:544-559.

Li LM, Timofeev I, Czosnyka M, Hutchinson PJA. The surgical approach to the management of increased intracranial pressure after traumatic brain injury. *Anesth Analg* 2010; 111; 736-748.

Lingsma HF, Roozenbeek B, Steyerberg EW et al. Early prognosis in traumatic brain injury: from prophecies to predictions. *Lancet Neurol* 2010; 9:543-554.

Maas AL, Stocchetti N, Bullock R. Moderate and severe traumatic brain injury in adults. *Lancet Neurol* 2008; 7: 728-741.

Smith M. Monitoring intracranial pressure in traumatic brain injury. *Anesth Analg* 2008; 106:240-248.

# 4 Fulminant Bacterial Meningitis

A 60-year-old woman presented initially to her family physician with a presumed sinusitis. She was treated with ciprofloxacin, but she did not complete a full antibiotic course. Over a matter of days she developed increasing headache and eventually nausea and vomiting. When she became less alert and confused, her husband brought her to the emergency room. On examination she was drowsy, but could follow a command when prompted. There was marked neck stiffness, but no other neurologic abnormalities were apparent. The emergency physician considered bacterial meningitis and proceeded with a CT scan that was normal. CSF showed 178 white blood cells per mm$^3$ with predominantly polynuclear cells, protein of 710 mg/dl, glucose of 7 mg/dl. Gram stain and blood cultures were negative. She was treated with dexamethasone, vancomycin, and ceftriaxone. Several days later she became much sleepier and eventually was unable to protect her airway, requiring intubation prior to transfer. On arrival to our neurosciences intensive care unit, she is opening her eyes to loud voice, only localizes to pain, and displays considerable neck stiffness.

The cranial nerve reflexes are normal, and there is no evidence of any focality on examination. CT scan shows a marked hydrocephalus and MR imaging shows marked gadolinium enhancement of the meninges (Figure 4.1).

## What do you do now?

One of the most dreaded clinical scenarios is a patient deteriorating from bacterial meningitis despite—what seems—appropriate antibiotic coverage.

Here are some useful facts.

*Streptococcus pneumonia* (or *pneumococcus*) is the most common cause of bacterial meningitis in adults. CSF gram stain and cultures, but also blood cultures readily and rapidly identify the bacteria in most cases. Infection with *Listeria monocytogenes* will have to be considered in elderly patients (over 60 years) and alcoholics. *Listeria monocytogenes* can be adequately eradicated by adding ampicillin (or ciprofloxacin) to an initial already broad empiric regimen with vancomycin and a third-generation cephalosporin.

There is compelling evidence that corticosteroids used early in the clinical course improve outcome, and most recent information shows a 10% reduction in mortality. There is uncertainty about the duration of administration, dose, and why corticosteroids reduce mortality (reducing brain edema, reducing inflammation and vasculitis, reducing the effects of associated septic shock).

Although a Cochrane analysis found no benefit, a more recent study found considerable benefit from corticosteroids (using historical controls) in meningitis caused by *Streptococcus pneumonia*. The data in meningococcal meningitis in adults remain uncertain, with one European study showing no benefit of corticosteroids.

Corticosteroids in patients with acute bacterial meningitis, however, remains common practice irrespective of the organism. The lingering concern is that reduction of the blood brain barrier permeability (as a result of reducing inflammation) may reduce penetration of antibiotics (particularly vancomycin). This effect may be overcome by additional use of rifampicin, but this drug is not often used. On the other hand, high-dose corticosteroids may have an effect on reducing or stabilizing diffuse cerebral edema. The main priorities of the initial treatment of bacterial meningitis are listed in Table 4.1.

So how can we explain the deterioration in our patient, and why is she not improving despite broad spectrum antibiotics? There are multiple causes of deterioration in fulminant bacterial meningitis and they are summarized in Table 4.2.

Several causes of deterioration are treatable. A major medical urgency is the development of a cerebral venous thrombosis of the cavernous sinus

TABLE 4.1 **First Priorities in Bacterial Meningitis**

Ceftriaxone 2 g IV every 12 hours

Vancomycin 20 mg/kg every 12 hours

Ampicillin 2 g every 6 hours

Dexamethasone 10 mg IV every 6 hours

Ventriculostomy with acute hydrocephalus

Mannitol 1-2 g/kg with acute brain edema

after a suppurative mastoiditis, which requires immediate intervention by an otolaryngologist. In other patients the appearance of epidural empyema—commonly associated with sinusitis and sinus surgery and mimicking bacterial meningitis—may be difficult to recognize and can be missed on a noncontrast CT scan of the brain (MRI is definitive). This is a neurosurgical emergency and requires craniotomy. Microabscesses are more difficult to treat, but when they rupture into the ventricles exploratory surgery may be needed. Abscesses in the posterior fossa are most concerning and also require neurosurgical drainage.

Acute hydrocephalus can be a major complication after bacterial meningitis (Figure 4.1). It is a manifestation of a more severe infection and occurs more often in comatose patients. The presence of hydrocephalus has been shown to be associated with higher fatality rates. Blockage may be at the foramina of Magendie and Luschka rather than at the pacchionian granulations. A ventricular drain is needed and could result in neurologic improvement.

TABLE 4.2 **Why Is the Patient with Bacterial Meningitis Deteriorating?**

| | |
|---|---|
| Wrong antibiotic | consider adding ampicillin for *Listeria monocytogenes* |
| Wrong diagnosis | consider epidural abscess |
| Wrong cause | consider nonconvulsive status epilepticus |
| Aggressive treatment needed | ventriculostomy, mannitol for brain edema, removal of cerebellar abscess after mastoiditis |
| Aggressive search for source needed | pneumonia, otitis media, mastoiditis, and sinusitis |

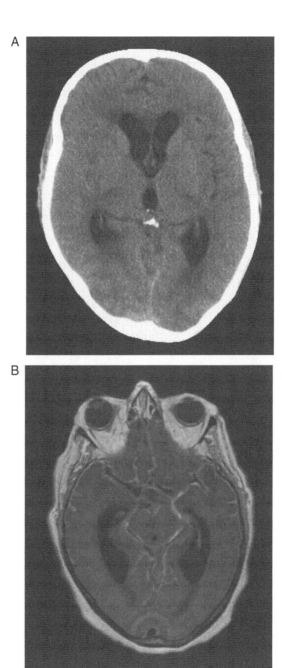

**FIGURE 4.1** CT scans shows early hydrocephalus (A) MRI shows dramatic meningeal enhancement. (B) Also, evidence of restricted diffusion in bilateral frontal temporal cortex indicative of additional laminar cortical necrosis due to infarction (C). MRA showed no evidence of arterial occlusions.

(*Continues*)

C

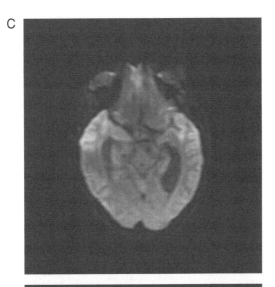

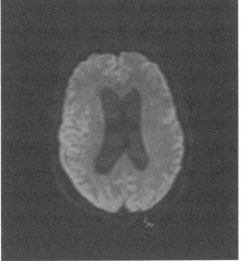

**FIGURE 4.1** *(Continued)*

Cerebral edema is mostly cytotoxic and can have a particularly rapid onset with subsequent loss of some brainstem reflexes. Immediate aggressive use of osmotic diuretics and high dose of intravenous corticosteroids may turn the tide, but many patients may progress further to loss of all brainstem reflexes.

Several causes of deterioration are untreatable. The development of ischemic lesions—as shown in our case—may be due to vasospasm, vasculitis, or vasculopathy. Cortical infarctions are common and widespread and rarely lead to swelling or mass effect. These abnormalities on CT scan are often mislabeled as "cerebritis." Vasculitis (or thrombotic vasculopathy) may lead to ischemia.

Brain injury can be rapid and permanent after an overwhelming infection. There is evidence that the brain may be an innocent bystander with leukocytes, macrophages, and microglia acting against invading bacteria, but at the same time releasing neurotoxic free radicals, proteases, cytokines, and other substances that result in neuronal cell death.

In our patient hydrocephalus was considered symptomatic despite the other areas of ischemic injury. A ventriculostomy was placed, and improvement of level of arousal occurred up to the point that extubation could be pursued. Nonetheless the patient remained severely impaired, uncommunicative, in need of gastrostomy and full nursing care. She died of a cardiac arrhythmia after the family had requested a do-not-resuscitate order.

Fulminant bacterial meningitis may be hard to treat effectively, and secondary manifestations (cerebral infarcts and hydrocephalus) may make recovery much less likely. Mortality in bacterial meningitis in the acute phase may be due to sepsis or multi-organ failure, but we suspect palliative care may be the most common reason of death in patients who remain comatose.

---

**KEY POINTS TO REMEMBER IN FULMINANT BACTERIAL MENINGITIS**

- Treat aggressively with corticosteroids and broad spectrum antibiotics as early as possible.
- MR imaging may explain neurologic condition.
- Patients may not improve due to cerebral infarcts or severe meningeal inflammation causing hydrocephalus.
- Cerebral edema may require osmotic diuretics and additional high dose corticosteroids.

## Further Reading

Assiri AM, Alamari FA, Zimmerman VA et al. Corticosteroid administration and outcome of adolescents and adults with acute bacterial meningitis: a meta analysis. *Mayo Clin Proc* 2009; 84: 403-409.

Brouwer MC, Heckenberg SGB, de Gans J et al. Nationwide implementation of adjunctive dexamethasone therapy for pneumococcal meningitis. *Neurology* 2010;75:1533-1539.

Kasanmoentalib ES, Brouwer MC, van der Ende A, van de Beek D. Hydrocephalus in adults with community-acquired bacterial meningitis. *Neurology* 2010;75:918-923.

Kim KS. Acute bacterial meningitis in infants and children. *Lancet Infect Dis* 2010; 10:32-42.

Muralidharan R, Rabinstein AA, Wijdicks EFM.Cervicomedullary injury after pneumococcal meningitis with brain edema. Arch Neurol. 2011;68:513-516.

Nudelman Y, Tunkel AR. Bacterial meningitis: epidemiology, pathogenesis and management update. *Drugs* 2009; 69:2577-2596.

Rosenstein NE, Perkins BA, Stephens DS, et al: Meningococcal disease. *N Engl J Med* 2001;344:1378-1388.

Van de Beek D, de Gans J, Tunkel AR, Wijdicks EFM. Community-acquired bacterial meningitis in adults. *N Engl J Med* 2006; 354:44-53.

# 5 Sorting Out and Treating Encephalitis

A 60-year-old woman was brought to the emergency department for evaluation of acute fever and confusion. She had psoriasis and rheumatoid arthritis, for which she was being treated with weekly doses of methotrexate and efalizumab and had recently received corticosteroids injections in her knees. Spiking fever had been first noticed one week before. Along with the fevers, she had been complaining of malaise and headache. Her primary internist suspected a urinary infection and had started her on levofloxacin two days before. She became more confused over the last 24 hours and was found in the neighbor's garage at night. We are called to examine her in the emergency department. She was tachycardic and had a temperature of 39.2° Celsius. She exhibited fluctuating level and content of consciousness. Her neck was rigid. Brainstem reflexes were preserved, and she had no lateralizing signs. CT scan showed low attenuation changes in the right temporal and insular regions (Figure 5.1 A and B).

*What do you do now?*

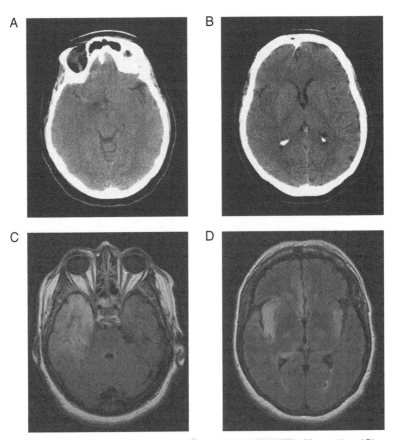

**FIGURE 5.1** Brain imaging in our patient with acute HSV-1 encephalitis. CT scan (A and B) showing low attenuation changes in the right temporal lobe and right insular region. Notice also the slightly hyperdense appearance in the Sylvian fissure, which may be confused for a fresh thrombus in the middle cerebral artery (A). The areas of brain swelling are much better visualized on the FLAIR sequence of the MRI (C and D), which also reveals the characteristic asymmetric bilaterality of the inflammation.

The diagnosis of encephalitis as a syndrome is relatively straightforward. Patients present with headache, fever, confusion, and, when more advanced, abnormal consciousness. Seizures (focal or more generalized) are a common manifestation. Examination may show neck stiffness or focal deficits, but there may be no localizing signs. In fact the diagnosis may not even be considered if the patient is seen early in the course and is just "confused". While the CT scan can be highly suggestive of certain forms of encephalitis (as illustrated by the temporal and insular areas of swelling in our patient with herpes simplex virus type 1 [HSV-1] encephalitis) (Figure 5.1), radiological changes are generally not characteristic of specific encephalitis etiologies. A brain MRI is far more helpful (Table 5.1). Cerebrospinal fluid (CSF) showing increased white blood cell count, and an increased protein concentration confirms the presence of encephalitis. A normal CSF strongly points towards alternative diagnoses (such as non-infectious limbic encephalitis).

Recognizing a clinical presentation consistent with the diagnosis of acute encephalitis is just the first step. Encephalitis can be infectious, postinfectious,

TABLE 5.1 **Causes of Acute Encephalitis with Characteristic Radiological Features**

| Cause | Characteristic radiological features |
|---|---|
| Herpes simplex virus type 1 | Inflammatory lesions in temporal lobes, insula, and operculum |
| Varicella herpes zoster | Multifocal infarctions and irregularities of arterial lumen<br>Cerebellitis in children |
| Cytomegalovirus | Ventriculitis (subependymal enhancement).<br>Brainstem inflammation |
| West Nile virus | Myelitis* |
| Tuberculosis | Basilar meningitis† |
| Fungal infections | Abscess formation** |
| Autoimmune limbic encephalitis | Inflammatory lesions in mesial temporal lobes |
| Acute disseminated encephalomyelitis | Bilateral white matter T2-hyperintense lesions.<br>Corpus callosum involvement |
| Progressive multifocal leukoencephalopathy (JC virus) | Bilateral, confluent T2-hyperintense lesions in temporo-occipital white matter with involvement of U fibers and cortical sparing |

* Presentation with acute flaccid paralysis may occur with or without radiological signs of myelitis.
† Also with fungal meningoencephalitis caused by Blastomycosis
** Aspergillus species is characterized by infarctions and hemorrhages

and noninfectious (Table 5.2). Autoimmune (paraneoplastic or not) and radiation-induced encephalitis are noninfectious examples. Defining the precise cause of the acute encephalitis is a much more difficult task that requires almost encyclopedic knowledge of neurological and infectious diseases, and working with a knowledgeable infectious disease consultant can be very helpful in these cases. Equally important is to narrow the differential diagnosis depending on the season, geographic area, specific exposures (including recent travel history) and risk factors.

Viral infection is the most common cause of acute encephalitis in adults. Epidemic outbreaks can be produced by the seasonal spread of arboviruses (i.e., viruses transmitted by arthropod vectors, such as mosquitoes). Most of these agents are constrained to specific geographical locations, but there are exceptions such as the West Nile virus or H1N1, which has been identified as a cause of outbreaks of encephalitis in all continents. Viral encephalitis can also be sporadic. Sporadic cases can occur in the immunocompetent and the immunodepressed patient.

HSV-1 is the most frequent cause of sporadic viral encephalitis in immunocompetent patients. HSV-1 encephalitis has a predilection for the temporal lobes, insula, and operculum. Consequently, it should be suspected when a febrile patient develops confusion or drowsiness associated with seizures or focal deficits referable to those locations. Aphasia, amnesia, hallucinations, agitation, visual field deficits and oral apraxia can be seen. When present, the typical distribution of swelling on brain MRI (Figure 5.1 C and D) strongly supports the diagnosis. Yet, the diagnosis should be established by confirming the presence of the virus in the CSF. Polymerase chain reaction (PCR) can detect HSV-1 DNA in the CSF with great sensitivity and specificity. If PCR is negative but the clinical-radiological presentation is suspicious for HSV-1 infection, the test should be repeated on a new CSF sample after 3–5 days.

Electroencephalography (EEG) should be performed in patients with HSV-1 encephalitis. It is not infrequent to see patients with encephalitis who exhibit fluctuating levels of alertness and awareness. In these cases we often pursue continuous EEG monitoring. Continuous EEG monitoring should also be considered in comatose patients with encephalitis. Nonconvulsive seizures are not uncommon but should be differentiated from periodic lateralized epileptiform discharges (PLEDs). Nonconvulsive

**TABLE 5.2   Main Causes of Acute Encephalitis, Diagnostic Test, and Principal Aspects of Management**

| Mechanism and etiology | Diagnostic test | Management principles |
|---|---|---|
| *Viral infections* | | |
| HSV-1 | CSF PCR | Acyclovir. Exclude seizures. |
| VZV | CSF PCR | Acyclovir +/- steroids |
| CMV | CSF PCR | Ganciclovir + foscarnet. Exclude HIV. |
| WNV | Serum IgM* | Supportive |
| Influenza | Viral culture, antigen, and PCR of respiratory tract specimen | Oseltamivir |
| Other arboviruses | CSF serology | Supportive. Exclude seizures. |
| JC virus (PML) | CSF PCR | Reverse anticoagulation HAART if HIV |
| HIV | CSF PCR (viral load) | HAART |
| Measles | Serum and CSF Ab PCR of nasopharynx, urine, brain | Ribavirin if life threatening |
| Mumps | Serum and CSF Ab | Supportive |
| Rabies | Serum and CSF Ab (if unvaccinated) IMF of viral antigen in nuchal biopsy Brain pathology | |
| *Bacterial infections †* | Serum antibodies CSF culture | Appropriate antibacterial drugs. |
| Mycobacterium tuberculosis | CSF AFB smear and culture CSF PCR (Gen-Probe Amplified)** | Isoniazid, rifampin, pyrazinamide, ethambutol plus steroids |
| Rickettsioses and Ehrlichioses | Serum Ab Morulae within PMN cells in blood smears (Ehrlichia only) | Doxycycline (add fluoroquinolone and rifampin if Coxiella) |
| Spirochetes Syphillis | Serum RPR, FTA-ABS CSF VDRL (specific but not sensitive) CSF FTA-ABS (sensitive but not specific) | Penicillin G |

*(Continues)*

TABLE 5.2   (Cont'd.)

| Mechanism and etiology | Diagnostic test | Management principles |
|---|---|---|
| Lyme | Serum and CSF Ab (ELISA + Western Blot) | Ceftriaxone |
| *Fungal infections ‡* | | |
| Aspergillosis | Serum antigen Tissue culture | Voriconazole or amphotericin B or caspofungin |
| Blastomycosis | Urine antigen Tissue culture | Amphotericin |
| Coccidiodomi-cosis | Serum and CSF Ab CSF culture | Fluconazole |
| Cryptococcosis | CSF Indian Ink stain Serum and CSF antigen Serum and CSF cultures | Amphotericin + flucytosine followed by fluconazole |
| Histoplasmosis | Urine and CSF antigen CSF Ab | Amphotericin B followed by fluconazole |
| *Protozoal infections* | | |
| Amebiasis | Serum Ab Brain biopsy (pathology and culture) | Trimethoprim-sulfamethoxazole + rifampin + keotconazole Check HIV serology |
| Malaria | Thick and thin blood Smears | Quinine. Avoid steroids. |
| Toxoplasmosis | Serum Ab MRI findings Response to therapy | Pyrimethamine + sulfadiazine or clindamycin Check HIV status |
| *Autoimmune encephalitis* | Paraneoplastic markers TPO Ab NMDA Receptor Ab | Immunotherapy (steroids, immuno-suppression, plasma exchange) Check for neoplasm |

Ab, antibodies; CMV, cytomegalovirus; CSF, cerebrospinal fluid; HAART, highly active antiretroviral therapy; HIV, human immunodeficiency virus; HSV-1, herpes simplex virus type 1; IMF, immunofluorescence; NMDA = N-methyl D-Aspartate; PML, Progressive multifocal leukoencephalopathy; PMN, polymorphonuclear; TPO, thyroid peroxidase; VZV, varicella-zoster virus; WNV, West Nile virus

*Serum antibodies are more sensitive than CSF antibodies.

† Bacterial infections that may present with acute encephalitis include Bartonella, Listeria (which characteristically causes a rhombencephalitis), Mycoplasma, and Tropherima whippeli.

** Sensitivity may not be optimal.

‡ Intrathecal amphotericin B may be necessary in severe cases.

seizures must be treated with antiepileptic drugs. When PLEDS are frequent or tend to become rhythmic, we also favor the use of antiepileptics to prevent seizures.

The role of brain biopsy has been relegated to very few selected cases thanks to the high yield of PCR. Brain biopsy in unexplained encephalitis is only considered once all noninvasive diagnostic alternatives have been exhausted and the patient continues to decline despite treatment with adequate doses of acyclovir. It is also advisable to search for other biopsy targets before invading the brain. Detailed physical examination with especial attention to the skin and lymph node chains; CT scans of chest, abdomen, and pelvis; and PET scan can deliver a more accessible site for tissue sampling. Brain biopsy should be guided by MRI findings, and we favor inclusion of a meningeal sample. When neuroimaging is unrevealing, the yield of random brain biopsy is much lower, but pathology may still be diagnostic in these cases. The most salient issue about the evaluation of unexplained encephalitis is how much of it may be without results—an intimidating assignment to say the least.

All patients with presumed acute encephalitis should be started immediately on intravenous acyclovir (10 mg/kg every 8 hours; longer intervals between doses in case of reduced glomerular filtration rate). This antiviral agent is the first choice for treating HSV-1, HSV-2, and varicella-zoster virus. Cytomegalovirus infection requires the combination of ganciclovir and foscarnet; these patients should also be tested for HIV infection. Ganciclovir and foscarnet are also the treatment for HSV-6 infection in immunosuppressed patients. No antiviral has proven effective against West Nile virus infection. HIV-infected patients must receive highly active antiretroviral therapy. In cases of progressive multifocal leukoencephalopathy (JC virus), the treatment consists of reversing immunosuppression. Main treatment measures for nonviral causes of encephalitis are summarized in Table 5.2.

Patients who develop severe brain swelling might require intracranial pressure monitoring. Intraparenchymal monitors are preferable when the ventricles are compressed by brain edema. Head of bed elevation and osmotic agents (mannitol, hypertonic saline) are the first step in cases of intracranial hypertension. The most severe cases may demand decompressive craniectomy. Corticosteroids do not have a role in the treatment of viral encephalitis.

The management of acute encephalitis may require admission to an intensive care unit. The major issues are recognition and treatment of seizures requiring video/EEG monitoring, mechanical ventilation in patients unable to protect the airway (due to abnormal consciousness or requirement of anesthetic drugs to control seizures or agitation), and treatment of brain swelling and medical complications. Even when the cause of the encephalitis is not treatable, aggressive supportive care increases the chance of a favorable outcome.

Our patient was started on intravenous acyclovir in the emergency department. An MRI of the brain (Figure 5.1 C and D) was obtained to delineate the degree of temporal lobe swelling before proceeding with lumbar puncture. The CSF contained 14 white blood cells (predominantly lymphocytes), a protein concentration of 58 mg/dL, and normal glucose level. Shortly after arrival to the ICU she was intubated because of progressive stupor and inability to protect the airway patency. Levofloxacin was stopped (it can reduce seizure threshold) and she was prophylactically started on intravenous levetiracetam. EEG demonstrated frequent periodic epileptiform discharges arising from the right temporal region but no electrographic seizures. Within hours we received confirmation that the PCR for HSV-1 was positive. She began to improve within the following 5 days. Two weeks later she was discharged home, where she continued recovering and completed a 21-day course of acyclovir. Her systemic immunosuppressive regimen was permanently stopped. Six months later she had regained full function.

> **KEY POINTS TO REMEMBER REGARDING SORTING OUT AND TREATING ACUTE ENCEPHALITIS**
>
> - Always consider the diagnosis of encephalitis in a febrile and confused patient, regardless of the presence of meningeal signs or focal deficits.
> - Start intravenous acyclovir in all patients with suspected viral encephalitis.
> - PCR for HSV-1 should be performed in all CSF samples of patients with presumed encephalitis. If PCR is negative but the diagnosis is still suspected (clinical or radiological localization to the temporal

lobes or insular/opercular region), acyclovir should be continued and PCR should be repeated after 3-5 days.

- MRI with gadolinium is the most informative neuroimaging modality for patients with suspected encephalitis.
- Every patient with HSV-1 encephalitis should have an EEG. In patients with fluctuating consciousness the option of continuous EEG monitoring should be considered to exclude nonconvulsive status epilepticus.

### Further Reading

Barnett GH, Ropper AH, Romeo J. Intracranial pressure and outcome in adult encephalitis. *J Neurosurg* 1988; 68:585-588.

Kastrup O, Wanke I, Maschke M. Neuroimaging of infections of the central nervous system. *Semin Neurol* 2008; 28:511-522.

McGrath N, Anderson NE, Croxson MC, Powell KF. Herpes simplex encephalitis treated with acyclovir: diagnosis and long term outcome. *J Neurol Neurosurg Psychiatry* 1997; 63:321-326.

Rosenfield MR, Dalmau J. Update on paraneoplastic and autoimmune disorders of the central nervous system. *Semin Neurol* 2010; 30:320-33.

Steiner I, Budka H, Chaudhuri A, Koskiniemi M, Sainio K, Salonen O, Kennedy PG. Viral meningoencephalitis: a review of diagnostic methods and guidelines for management. *Eur J Neurol* 2010; 17:999-1009.

Tunkel AR, Glaser CA, Bloch KC, Sejvar JJ, Marra CM, Roos KL, Hartman BJ, Kaplan SL, Scheld WM, Whitley RJ; Infectious Diseases Society of America. The management of encephalitis: clinical practice guidelines by the Infectious Diseases Society of America. *Clin Infect Dis* 2008; 47:303-327.

Whitley RJ, Gnann JW. Viral encephalitis: familiar infections and emerging pathogens. *Lancet* 2002, 359:507-513.

# Respiratory Support in Acute Neuromuscular Respiratory Failure

A 21-year-old woman presented to our emergency department complaining of low back pain for the last two days, tingling in her legs since the previous afternoon, and difficulty urinating since the previous evening. Over the preceding hours she had noticed progressive weakness in her legs. On initial evaluation she had weakness in both legs, which was mild proximally and moderate distally. Her deep tendon reflexes were absent in both legs and decreased in both arms. Sensory examination was unremarkable. She had no signs of oropharyngeal weakness or ventilatory problems. Arterial blood gases revealed neither hypoxia nor hypercapnia. Chest film was normal. She was admitted to our intensive care unit for close monitoring.

Early the following morning we notice she is much weaker. She can hardly activate her iliopsoas muscles and cannot move her legs. Her arms can barely stay up against gravity. She is now completely arreflexic. Restless and tachypneic, she reports difficulty breathing and can only speak a few words at the time because of her breathlessness.

**What do you do now?**

ntubation is imminent, but what causes the patient's shortness of breath?

An acute neuromuscular disorder should be suspected in any patient with acute respiratory failure who presents with mixed hypoxia and hypercapnea or predominant hypercapnea with signs of oropharyngeal and appendicular muscle weakness. The most likely causes are Guillain-Barré syndrome or myasthenia gravis. Myopathy or a previously undiagnosed motor neuron disease are less frequent but possible considerations. Patients with neuromuscular respiratory failure have a characteristic presentation. They are dyspneic, tachypneic, and tachycardic. Restlessness is a very common feature, inability to speak in full sentences (staccato speech) and diaphoresis (typically seen as sweat on the forehead) denote their great difficulty to breathe. Patients with oropharyngeal weakness will have a weak cough, nasal voice, and problems handling oral secretions. Recruitment of accessory muscles can be visible on inspection, but it is best noted by palpating the sternocleidomastoid muscles. Yet, the hallmark of neuromuscular respiratory failure is the presence of paradoxical breathing pattern, an inward rather than the normal outward movement of the abdominal wall with each inspiration.

These clinical manifestations are due to failure of the breathing mechanics eventually leading to insufficient ventilation. In a nutshell it goes as follows. Failure of the diaphragm (large component) and intercostal muscles (small component) to lift the ribcage can only be partly compensated by other muscles attached to the ribcage (accessory muscles). The abdominal muscles only assist with coughing and expiration. Poor lung expansion leads to reduced air flow and alveolar collapse. Atelectasis causes hypoxemia and, eventually, hypoventilation results in hypercapnia. Aspiration due to coexisting oropharyngeal weakness may worsen gas exchange even more. The inadequate physiologic compensatory response consists of increasing the respiratory frequency, while the tidal volumes remain small. So, when physicians enter the room they may see a patient visibly struggling to breathe, sitting up in bed and maintaining only marginal pulse oximeter values (oxygen saturations in the low 90s) despite increasing oxygen requirements. Hypercapnia occurs later in acute cases, but may be seen early in patients with exacerbations of chronic neuromuscular disorders.

Bedside spirometry to gauge forced vital capacity, and maximal inspiratory and expiratory pressures, arterial blood gases, and a chest X-ray should complement physical examination in the initial evaluation of these patients. Be sure to coach patients carefully before spirometry testing and check if they can satisfactorily seal the mouth piece of the spirometer with their lips before moving forward with the test. When the results are much poorer than expected—based on the physical exam and the blood gases—poor technique, insufficient mouth sealing, or suboptimal effort are the most frequent explanations.

When after this initial assessment your diagnosis is indeed neuromuscular respiratory failure, the next steps are deciding whether the patient needs mechanical ventilation and what is the most likely cause of the weakness. Both of these priorities are closely related. The urgency of action and the type of mechanical ventilation to be chosen will depend on the neuromuscular disorder being treated. Being able to establish the neuromuscular diagnosis is not only crucial to select optimal treatment, but also carries major prognostic implications. Patients with acute neuromuscular respiratory failure of unclear cause after extensive evaluations—a situation we encounter in more than 10% of all cases admitted to the ICU with acute neuromuscular respiratory failure—rarely recover well despite aggressive respiratory treatment.

Guillain-Barré syndrome (GBS) and myasthenic crisis are the most common causes of acute neuromuscular respiratory failure. Although these two immunological disorders are similar in some aspects, the ideal respiratory management differs substantially between the two. Patients with GBS can get worse very fast and when they do, they often have manifestations of dysautonomia, such as rapid swings in blood pressure and cardiac arrhythmias. Also, once they have developed ventilatory impairment their course toward full-blown respiratory failure is unstoppable. Those patients should be intubated without delay before they reach their nadir because they may develop sudden respiratory arrest and emergency intubation can trigger severe cardiocirculatory complications. Spirometry results can be confidently used to guide the timing of elective intubation in GBS (Table 6.1). Other clinical pointers are shown in Table 6.2.

However the approach in patients worsening from myasthenia gravis can be different. Patients that are approaching a myasthenic crisis may benefit

**TABLE 6.1** **Bedside Respiratory Tests Predicting Need for Mechanical Ventilation in GBS**

| Parameter | Normal value | Critical value* |
|---|---|---|
| Forced vital capacity | 40-70 ml/kg | 20 ml/kg |
| Maximal inspiratory pressure | Men: > -100 cmH$_2$O<br>Women: > -70 cmH$_2$O | -30 cmH$_2$O |
| Maximal expiratory pressure | Men: > 200 cmH$_2$O<br>Women: > 140 cmH$_2$O | 40 cmH$_2$O |

*Best remembered as the 20-30-40 rule.*

*[handwritten: FVC 20 ml/kg; INSP. -30 cm H₂O; EXP. 40 cm H₂O; "20-30-40" rule]*

from early noninvasive ventilatory support with bilevel positive airway pressure (BiPAP). Contrary to GBS and other acute or chronic nerve disorders respiratory muscles of patients with myasthenic gravis develop progressive but still reversible fatigability before they fail. When aided by BiPAP, these muscles can sustain adequate ventilation longer, thus allowing time for immuno-modulatory therapy to become effective. If started timely, BiPAP can avert intubation and prevent pulmonary complications (atelectasis and pneumonia). However, one should not wait to start BiPAP. Once patients become hypercapnic—an indication that the ventilatory muscles have already failed—noninvasive ventilation is very likely to be unsuccessful. Although bedside spirometry results are often used in myasthenic crisis, they are less reliable indicators of the need of mechanical ventilation than in GBS.

**TABLE 6.2** **Clinical Findings that Predict Rapid Worsening and Need for Intubation in Patients with Acute Neuromuscular Respiratory Weakness**

Pooling secretions due to oropharyngeal weakness

Increased work of breathing and restlessness

Rapidly progressive muscle weakness

Increasing oxygen requirements

Failure to improve with BiPAP*

Aspiration or major atelectasis on chest X-ray

Evidence of respiratory infection

*BiPAP is not recommended for patients with Guillain-Barré syndrome.*

Our patient had an axonal type of GBS. We intubated our patient immediately that morning and in a matter of hours she progressed further and was completely paralyzed by her disease. During her ICU admission she developed various manifestations of severe dysautonomia, including a short period of asystole during tracheal suctioning and sudden hypertensive surges and hypotensive plunges (see also chapter 23). Despite the extreme severity of her disease at nadir, she recovered full function within the following year.

Decision making in acute neuromuscular respiratory failure requires good judgment. In myasthenia gravis, early use of BiPAP may prevent the need for intubation and prolonged mechanical ventilation. In GBS, the neuromuscular respiratory failure may progress very rapidly and become extremely difficult to manage or even lead to a fatal outcome if physicians hesitate to intubate.

---

**KEY POINTS TO REMEMBER REGARDING RESPIRATORY SUPPORT FOR ACUTE NEUROMUSCULAR RESPIRATORY FAILURE**

- Paradoxical breathing is the most characteristic sign of neuromuscular respiratory failure.
- Identifying the neuromuscular cause of the ventilatory failure is essential to formulate the best plan for respiratory management.
- Patients with GBS should be intubated electively when they develop their first signs of ventilatory failure (i.e. before hypoxemia and certainly before hypercapnia).
- Patients with myasthenic crisis are best treated with noninvasive ventilation (BiPAP) if this support is initiated before the development of hypercapnia.

---

Further Reading

Cabrera Serrano M, Rabinstein AA. Causes and outcomes of acute neuromuscular respiratory failure. *Arch Neurol* 2010; 67:1089-1094.

Lawn ND, Fletcher DD, Henderson RD, Wolter TD, Wijdicks EFM. Anticipating mechanical ventilation in Guillain-Barré syndrome. *Arch Neurol* 2001; 58:893-898.

Mehta S. Neuromuscular disease causing acute respiratory failure. *Respir Care* 2006; 51:1016-1021.

Rabinstein AA, Wijdicks EFM. Warning signs of imminent respiratory failure in neurological patients. *Semin Neurol* 2003; 23:97-104.

Seneviratne J, Mandrekar J, Wijdicks EFM, Rabinstein AA. Noninvasive ventilation in myasthenic crisis. *Arch Neurol* 2008; 65:54-58.

Walgaard C, Lingsma HF, Ruts L, Drenthen J, van Koningsveld R, Garssen MJ, van Doorn PA, Steyerberg EW, Jacobs BC. Prediction of respiratory insufficiency in Guillain-Barré syndrome. *Ann Neurol* 2010; 67:781-787.

Wijdicks EFM, Henderson RD, McClelland RL. Emergency intubation for respiratory failure in Guillain-Barré syndrome. *Arch Neurol* 2003; 60:947-948.

# Endovascular Recanalization in Acute Stroke

A 53-year-old man with history of hypertension and atrial fibrillation previously treated with ablation and currently not anticoagulated presented to an emergency department after developing sudden onset of speech difficulties and right-sided weakness. Initial head CT scan showed no acute abnormalities. The patient had no contraindications for thrombolysis. He was treated with 0.9 mg/kg of intravenous recombinant tissue plasminogen activator (rt-PA) starting 2 hours after symptom onset. He was then transferred to our hospital for further assessment.

On arrival to our emergency department he is alert, globally aphasic, and has a right hemianopia, left gaze preference and right hemiplegia. His NIH stroke scale sum score is 22.

**What do you do now?**

ntravenous thrombolysis with rt-PA within 4.5 hours after symptom onset is the only recanalization therapy supported by solid evidence and currently considered standard of care. However, commonly we encounter patients with severe deficits who fail to improve after intravenous thrombolysis or have contraindications for this treatment. In these cases we and many other centers around the world consider the option of attempting endovascular recanalization. Endovascular recanalization can be achieved by infusing drugs or using mechanical devices. Only a pharmacological approach has been shown effective in a randomized controlled trial. This trial (PROACT-II) tested intra-arterial pro-urokinase injected in the clot within 6 hours of stroke symptoms. This drug is no longer manufactured, and intra-arterial rt-PA is used instead. Currently, devices for mechanical embolectomy are used first when attempting endovascular recanalization while intra-arterial thrombolysis has become more often an adjuvant therapy. It is true that using whatever it takes to open an occluded major artery is justified because whether or not recanalization is achieved strongly predicts outcome in these patients. Yet it is unfortunate that the strategy of mechanical embolectomy was not evaluated more rigorously prior to their aggressive marketing. The field of endovascular stroke treatment is in flux, influenced by the newest (ingenious) device and without a consensus among "neurointerventionalists" on what should be the best practices. Randomized trials seem unlikely to be completed soon. Yet, there is a good reason to be optimistic that the emergent care of patients with severe ischemic stroke due to a major intracranial vessel occlusion may improve substantially in the future.

The major question, however, is what patients should be considered good candidates for endovascular therapies. We have incorporated CT angiogram and CT perfusion in our decision model to determine who has the best opportunity of improving after recanalization. Our selection criteria are summarized in Table 7.1.

We favor endovascular recanalization when there is a major intracranial vessel occlusion (M1 or large M2 branch of the middle cerebral artery, extracranial or intracranial carotid artery, dominant vertebral artery, or basilar artery) along with radiological evidence of ischemic penumbra (more than 25% mismatch between the area of perfusion abnormality and the

TABLE 7.1 **Conditions to be Met by Candidates for Endovascular Recanalization Therapy for Acute Ischemic Stroke**

Severe, incapacitating neurological deficits

Large intracranial vessel occlusion

Presence of radiological penumbra

    Failure of intravenous thrombolysis*

    or

    Contraindications for intravenous thrombolysis, such as:

        Time from symptom onset > 4.5 hours

        Recent surgery

        History of intracranial hemorrhage

        Active anticoagulation

Good prestroke level of function

Good rehabilitation potential

*We occasionally proceed directly with endovascular recanalization attempt in cases of carotid artery occlusion or basilar artery occlusion.

area of reduced blood volume) in the absence of a large infarction (as estimated by the area of reduced cerebral blood volume). We tend to estimate the region of ischemic penumbra by the mismatch between the mean transit time and the cerebral blood volume. This model is more sensitive than comparing cerebral blood flow versus cerebral blood volume, but we realize it is less specific and might overestimate the area of salvageable tissue. Other groups use MRI scans (diffusion/perfusion mismatch) for patient selection. The two imaging techniques appear to be fairly comparable for decision-making.

Large areas of infarction (by restricted diffusion on MRI or reduced cerebral blood volume on CT perfusion scan) before the intervention strongly predict postprocedural bleeding. Therefore, patients with these findings should not be considered safe candidates for reperfusion therapy, and the rates of symptomatic hemorrhage may be as high as 50–80%. (To put this rate in perspective, among all patients, the rate of symptomatic intracranial bleeding after endovascular stroke therapy is approximately 10% regardless of the strategy used.)

The number of devices approved for mechanical removal of intracranial clots is increasing. Clot retrievers (MERCI device) and suction/separator catheters (PENUMBRA system) are currently most often used, but retrievable intracranial stents hold great promise. The selection of these devices varies (mostly determined by the personal preference of the neurointerventionalist), and more than one type may be tried in the same case. Intraarterial rt-PA is frequently infused when devices fail to open the vessel or achieve only partial opening.

Studies publishing the experience with the use of certain devices have reported rates of recanalization in excess of 80%. It remains to be shown whether this can be reproduced in most practices. Of those patients who recanalize, a substantial proportion experience improved deficits but only a minority regains good function. While it is true that this can be explained because these patients start with large areas of ischemia and severe symptoms, there may be other factors apart from recanalization that affect the chances of recovery. For instance, it has been proposed that doing the intervention under general anesthesia rather than conscious sedation might worsen the chances of favorable functional recovery. Other factors associated with worse prognosis after endovascular stroke therapy are listed in Table 7.2.

TABLE 7.2 **Indicators of Poor Prognosis after Acute Endovascular Stroke Therapy**

Lack of recanalization or persistent distal occlusion

Worse initial stroke severity

Large area of diffusion restriction or reduced CBV before the intervention

Absence of large radiological penumbra before the intervention

Poor collateral arterial supply

Internal carotid artery occlusion

Postprocedural intracranial hemorrhage

*(Continues)*

## TABLE 7.2  (Cont'd.)

*Older age*

*Major comorbidities*

*General anesthesia*

*Atrial fibrillation*

*Diabetes mellitus*

*Admission hyperglycemia*

CBV, cerebral blood volume.
Probable associations in italics

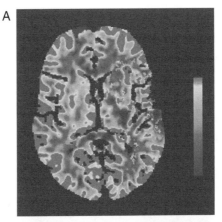

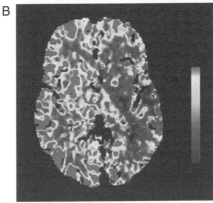

**FIGURE 7.1**  CT perfusion revealing a large mismatch between the areas of reduced cerebral blood volume (A) and decreased cerebral blood flow (B).

Our patient represents a common clinical scenario—major deficit despite IV rt-PA and opportunity of an endovascular intervention. After confirming the presence of persistent left middle cerebral artery occlusion and a large area of ischemic penumbra in the left middle cerebral artery territory (Figure 7.1), the patient was taken to the angiography suite. The intervention started 3 hours and 30 minutes after symptom onset. Large amounts of clot were suctioned and the patient also received 6 mg of intra-arterial rt-PA. Recanalization was achieved after 80 minutes (Figure 7.2).

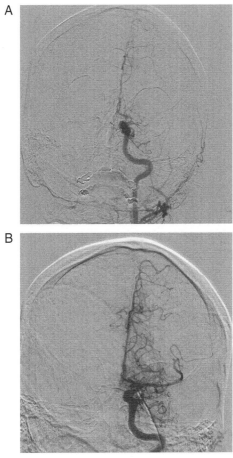

**FIGURE 7.2** A) Preprocedural cerebral catheter angiogram showing occlusion of the left middle cerebral artery. B) Recanalization after endovascular intervention.

The patient evolved favorably over the following days. He was initially discharged to the inpatient rehabilitation unit and then went home 21 days after the stroke. By that time, he had regained functional independence with mild residual expressive dysphasia, a right visual field deficit, and mild to moderate right hemiparesis. He could walk with a cane and climb a flight of stairs without assistance. His NIH stroke scale sum score was 5. Three months later he had mild residual deficits (modified Rankin score of 2). His brain infarctions are shown in Figure 7.3.

As illustrated by this case, we have seen patients improving substantially after complete (Figure 7.4) or even partial endovascular recanalization. Other patients fail to get any better, and some others develop hemorrhagic conversion or a large intracerebral hematoma. Large territorial infarcts may go on to develop swelling, resulting in more complex decisions (discussed in chapter 8). In fact, the care of patients with a major ischemic stroke has become a specialized field, and there is proof that these patients do better when admitted to stroke units or neurosciences intensive care units manned by specialized teams.

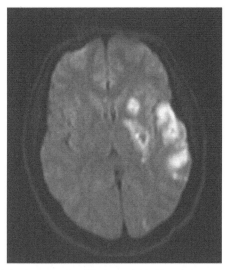

**FIGURE 7.3** Brain infarctions on MRI (diffusion-weighted imaging sequence).

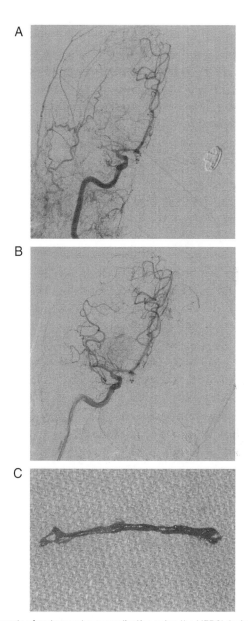

**FIGURE 7.4** Example of endovascular recanalization using the MERCI device.
A) Preprocedural cerebral catheter angiogram showing occlusion of the right middle
cerebral artery. B) Recanalization of the artery following endovascular intervention.
C) Photograph of the clot retrieved from this patient by the MERCI device.

**Further Reading**

Baker WL, Colby JA, Tongbram V et al. Neurothrombectomy devices for the treatment of acute ischemic stroke: state of the evidence. *Ann Intern Med* 2011; 154:243-252.

Brinjinkji W, Rabinstein AJ, Kallmes DF et al. Patient outcomes with endovascular embolectomy therapy for acute ischemic stroke: A study of the national inpatient sample 2006-2008. *Stroke* 2011; in press.

Castaño C, Dorado L, Guerrero C et al. Mechanical thrombectomy with the Solitaire AB device in large artery occlusions of the anterior circulation: a pilot study. *Stroke* 2010; 41:1836-1840.

Furlan A, Higashida R, Wechsler L et al. Intra-arterial prourokinase for acute ischemic stroke. The PROACT II study: a randomized controlled trial. PROlyse in Acute Cerebral Thromboembolism. *JAMA* 1999; 282:2003-2011.

Hallevi H, Barreto AD, Liebeskind DS et al; UCLA Intra-Arterial Therapy Investigators, Grotta JC, Savitz SI. Identifying patients at high risk for poor outcome after intra-arterial therapy for acute ischemic stroke. *Stroke* 2009; 40:1780-1785.

Molina CA. Reperfusion therapies for acute ischemic stroke: current pharmacological and mechanical approaches. *Stroke*. 2011;42:S16-S19.

Penumbra Pivotal Stroke Trial Investigators. The penumbra pivotal stroke trial: safety and effectiveness of a new generation of mechanical devices for clot removal in intracranial large vessel occlusive disease. *Stroke* 2009; 40:2761-2768.

Smith WS, Sung G, Saver J et al. Mechanical thrombectomy for acute ischemic stroke: final results of the Multi Merci trial. *Stroke* 2008; 39:1205-1212.

Wintermark M, Meuli R, Browaeys P et al. Comparison of CT perfusion and angiography and MRI in selecting stroke patients for acute treatment. *Neurology* 2007; 68: 694-697.

# 8  Decompressive Craniectomy in Acute Stroke

A 48-year-old man was found by his wife on the bathroom floor. His speech was slurred, and the left side was weak. In an outside hospital, he was found to have profound left-sided weakness and neglect. The NIH Stroke Scale sum score was reportedly 17. A CT showed a right hyperdense MCA sign, and CTA showed bilaterally occluded carotid arteries. He received intravenous tPA. No endovascular intervention was available. The patient was transferred, and on arrival he does not open his eyes to pain, he has minimally reactive 4 mm pupils, but corneal reflexes are intact. There is a forced eye deviation to the right. He is localizing to pain only on the right side. Left arm and leg are flaccid and do not move after a noxious stimulus. He has Cheyne-Stokes breathing, but there are no marked hypoxemic episodes, and he seems to protect his airway well. He has atrial fibrillation, but with a normal ventricular response, and blood pressure is consistently within the normal range. A repeat CT scan shows an evolving infarct involving the right frontal, parietal, basal ganglia, and caudate nucleus areas. A significant midline shift is noted.

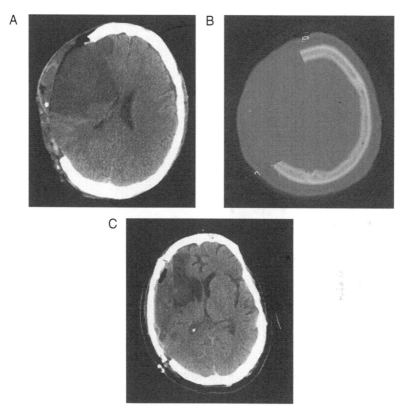

**FIGURE 8.1** CT scan (A, B) showing extensive decompressive craniectomy (with duraplasty using bovine pericardial graft) for swollen hemispheric infarct. Replacement of bone flap seen on repeat CT scan 6 months later (C).

Doing nothing knowing the patient will lapse into coma is not an option in a relatively young person. Further swelling of a major territorial infarct can be anticipated in acute carotid artery occlusion, and often these are patients who deteriorate beyond drowsiness. Medical management with osmotic diuretics is often ineffective, and patients may worsen rather quickly. Decompressive hemicraniectomy may result in a recovery that could potentially be meaningful for the patient. Yet, when it comes to the question of creating space to swell, preemptive removal of half the skull at the site of a newly developing hemispheric infarct may be perceived as overly aggressive. Responsible physicians will have to weigh in expected quality of life, social factors such as support from family members, age, and comorbidity.

What do we know from clinical trials? In a recent pooled analysis of (incompleted) randomized trials the natural history of a large hemispheric infarct (i.e., occlusion of the middle cerebral artery or carotid artery occlusion) was death in 60% and severe disability in nearly 30%. Comparison of the "natural history" with the outcome of patients undergoing decompressive hemicraniectomy remains seriously flawed due to unavoidable less aggressive care in non-surgically treated patients.

There is however good data showing that decompressive hemicraniectomy may be a life-saving procedure. There are also good physiologic arguments for decompressive surgery when performed early in the process. Apart from preventing permanent brainstem injury from direct compression, a reduction of intracranial pressure—even if marginally elevated—may improve cerebral blood flow and brain tissue oxygenation. These effects could allow an improved functional recovery in a proportion of survivors, as observed in recent trials.

The questions are: can we identify the best candidates for decompressive craniectomy, and what should trigger surgery in patients with hemispheric infarcts? Should this large hemicraniectomy be offered to all patients regardless of age, level of consciousness, involvement of vascular territories, or hemispheric dominance? Could early MRI predict clinical deterioration or does it only predict radiologic worsening? We have no satisfactory answers to most of these questions. Some criteria to help in a decision are shown in Table 8.1.

Timing of surgery remains undefined, but clinical deterioration is needed for most neurosurgeons to act. More than a few neurosurgeons confronted

Age less than 60 years
Rehabilitation opportunities
Patient able to cope with severe handicap
No major comorbidity
Any clinical deterioration in consciousness and need for intubation
Anticipated or documented multiple territorial involvement
Early (< 24 h) evidence of mass effect on CT scan

with a patient with a massive swollen infarct will still have to be convinced there is benefit to be gained from surgery. Other uncertainties are the technique of decompression—size of craniectomy, removal of additional bone from the squamous part of the temporal bone, extent of the durotomy, removal of the temporalis muscle, among other options.

What did we do? Our patient underwent decompressive hemicraniectomy and developed considerable swelling outside the skull but without clinical deterioration (Figure 8.1A, B). It is easy to imagine it would have caused severe deterioration with a swollen ischemic mass in a smaller confined space. Six months later (Figure 8.1C) his functional outcome was not truly favorable despite his being able to ambulate with a cane and being able to take oral intake. He had impaired judgment, was barely interactive, had depressed mood, impaired orientation, difficulty expressing his needs, and required assistance with bathing, toileting, and transfers from bed to chair. In summary, his outcome 6 months later can hardly be called satisfactory, and we do not know if more improvement is expected over time.

Medical management of large hemisphere strokes has been frustrating. Part of the problem is that these infarctions are complicated by an unrelenting swelling unresponsive to usual "antiedema" therapy. Mannitol and hypertonic saline have been inadequately evaluated for the treatment of ischemic brain edema, although clinical empirical experience is mixed, with some patients improving clinically and others progressing to development of brainstem involvement. Hyperventilation in patients intubated for airway protection has not been studied systematically, may negatively impact on cerebral oxygenation, and thus cannot be recommended except for very brief periods. Therapeutic hypothermia—using cooling devices—is increasing but its value in this clinical situation is just being studied in controlled clinical trials.

The main principle of neurocritical management is to avoid further brain injury. Therefore, attention should be directed to maintain adequate intravascular volume (hydrate with 0.9% saline avoiding hypotonic solutions and excessively positive fluid balance), treat fever (using a cooling device if necessary), treat aspiration pneumonitis (with broad-spectrum antibiotics until cultures are known), provide deep venous thrombosis prophylaxis (subcutaneous heparin three times a day) and control blood pressure (systolic blood pressure less than 180 mg and diastolic less than 105 mg). Swallowing precautions are needed and most patients need nasogastric feeding.

A guarded attitude toward these massive cerebral infarcts is understandable, but surgical treatment may be beneficial in some cases. There are some patients who are grateful for such aggressive care. But it is very difficult to know who those patients will be.

---

**KEY POINTS TO REMEMBER REGARDING DECOMPRESSIVE CRANIECTOMY IN ACUTE STROKE**

- Middle cerebral artery territory infarcts may be due to acute carotid occlusion and such infarcts may become more extensive and particularly severe.
- Malignant hemispheric swelling occurs in 30% of patients with large vessel occlusion.
- Medical management with osmotic diuretics is often unhelpful.
- Decompressive craniectomy should be considered in patients < 60 years, with mass effect on CT scan and evidence of early neurologic decline.
- Decompressive craniectomy may reduce mortality, but neurologic morbidity is considerable and an issue of utmost importance to address with proxy.

---

Further Reading

Bardutzky J, Schwab S. Antiedema therapy in ischemic stroke. *Stroke* 2007; 38: 3084-3094.

Huttner HB, Schwab S. Malignant middle cerebral artery infarction: clinical characteristics, treatment strategies, and future perspectives. *Lancet Neurol* 2009; 8:949-958.

Maramattom BV, Bahn MM, Wijdicks EFM. Which patient fares worse after early deterioration due to swelling from hemispheric stroke? *Neurology* 2004; 63: 2142-2145.

Rabinstein AA, Mueller-Kronast N, Maramattom BV et al. Factors predicting prognosis after decompressive hemicraniectomy for hemispheric infarction. *Neurology* 2006; 67:891-893.

Staykov D, Gupta R. Hemicraniectomy in malignant middle cerebral artery infarction. *Stroke.* 2011;42:513-516.

Thomalla G, Hartmann F, Juettler E. Prediction of malignant middle cerebral artery infarction by magnetic resonance imaging within 6 hours of symptom onset: a prospective multicenter observational study. *Ann Neurol* 2010; 68:435-445.

Vahedi K, Hofmeijer J, Juettler E et al; DECIMAL, DESTINY, and HAMLET investigators. Early decompressive surgery in malignant infarction of the middle cerebral artery: a pooled analysis of three randomized controlled trials. *Lancet Neurol* 2007; 6:215-222.

Wijdicks EFM. Management of massive hemispheric cerebral infarct: Is there a ray of hope? *Mayo Clin Proc* 2000; 75:945-952.

# Neurological Worsening After Subarachnoid Hemorrhage

A 44-year-old woman presented to the emergency department after having a thunderclap headache. Her past medical history was only significant for current smoking. Her neurological examination was normal, and she was alert (World Federation of Neurological Surgeons grade I). Head CT scan revealed diffuse hemorrhage in the subarachnoid cisterns with some blood in the lateral ventricles, which had preserved size (modified Fisher grade 4) (Figure 9.1A). She was admitted to our neurosciences ICU for further care.

Three hours later she became increasingly drowsy. Her blood pressure trended upward, and she developed sinus bradycardia. Her neurological examination still showed no focal deficits, but upward eye movements were limited. Repeat head CT scan confirmed the suspected hydrocephalus (Figure 9.1B). She improved back to normal after placement of a ventriculostomy catheter.

The following morning she underwent endovascular coiling of her ruptured anterior communicating artery aneurysm without complications. She remained well until postbleeding day 5, when she was noticed to be slightly confused. Mean blood flow velocities on transcranial Doppler had increased by 30% compared with the previous day, with maximal velocities in the 180 cm/s range. Her mild confusion fluctuated over the following 24 hours. Now, examining the patient on postbleeding day 6, she is at times restless and at times drowsy. Although still oriented to her situation when fully awake, she cannot answer minimally complex questions and gets easily distracted. Motor examination reveals a left pronator drift for the first time. Her ventriculostomy is draining well. She is febrile (38.6 degrees Celsius) and actually has been having high temperatures for several hours with poor response to acetaminophen. She is mildly hypertensive and has been polyuric overnight. Laboratory tests show no leukocytosis and a serum sodium concentration of 132 mmol/L (from 136 mmol/L the day before).

**What do you do now?**

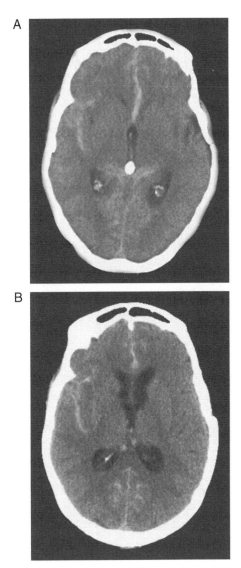

**FIGURE 9.1** A) Initial head CT scan showing SAH with aneurysmal pattern and some blood layering in the lateral ventricles consistent with a modified Fisher scale grade 4. B) Follow-up CT scan nearly 4 hours later shows hydrocephalus.

Patients with an aneurysmal subarachnoid hemorrhage (aSAH) often appear deceptively stable. They may "look great" only to acutely or gradually decline into a much worse neurologic state. The very moment when changes in neurologic condition occur are sometimes difficult to pinpoint (as with cerebral vasospasm) but in other instances changes are overwhelmingly clear (as with rebleeding). When caring for a patient with aSAH with worsening neurological condition, the differential diagnosis to be considered will also depend on the time from aneurysm rupture. This is clearly demonstrated by this patient, who declined early due to hydrocephalus and later because of cerebral vasospasm.

The major risks to the patient on the first day after aneurysmal rupture are rebleeding and acute hydrocephalus. It is hard to overlook a rebleeding because the clinical changes are dramatic. The patient suddenly becomes stuporous or comatose and the altered consciousness is accompanied by severe hypertension, tachypnea (or apnea), and tachycardia (or brief asystole). Motor responses change, and extensor posturing (mimicking a seizure to the untrained observer) may occur. In comatose patients with a poor grade aSAH, rebleeding may cause loss of pupillary and corneal reflexes, and nursing staff may see fresh blood in the ventriculostomy bag. This catastrophic event is markedly different from the presentation of hydrocephalus. Instead, as hydrocephalus develops patients become progressively less interactive, then drowsier, and finally unresponsive. While this progression may be rapid, it is not sudden, and alarms do not go off as patients only are mildly hypertensive and bradycardic. While patients are still arousable the only physical sign may be restricted eye movements in the vertical plane caused by the pressure of the expanded third ventricle over the tectum of the brainstem. Given the paucity of clinical clues, the recognition of acute hydrocephalus remains a challenge for physicians outside the neurosciences and many do not appreciate the dilated ventricles on CT scan.

Delayed vasospasm occurs days later, typically starting 3 to 5 days after the hemorrhage to reach a peak around day 7 before resolving by days 10 to 12. Contrary to a common assumption of trainees, the first manifestation of vasospasm is usually not a focal deficit. Instead, diminished alertness and lucidity tend to be the presenting symptoms of this complication. Patients developing cerebral vasospasm are often febrile and have developed hyponatremia, which are factors that can also diminish alertness. Consequently the diagnosis of symptomatic cerebral vasospasm is far from straightforward, and good clinical judgment and experience are necessary to recognize it. Some patients are at higher risk for ischemic damage from cerebral vasospasm after aSAH and these risk factors are listed in Table 9.1. Useful modalities for the screening of vasospasm and diagnosis of delayed cerebral ischemia are summarized in Table 9.2.

Transcranial Doppler (TCD) is useful to monitor for cerebral vasospasm, especially when trends from serial measurements are documented. We suspect cerebral vasospasm when the mean blood flow velocity in the M1 segment of the middle cerebral artery exceeds 120 cm/s and consider it severe when this measurement is greater than 200 cm/s. We have been increasingly using a combination of CT angiogram and CT perfusion in patients with suspected vasospasm. Conventional angiography is reserved for patients who are refractory to medical therapy and might be candidates for endovascular treatment. However, all these techniques have limitations. Cerebral vasospasm is primarily caused by endothelial dysfunction and involves first and foremost the microcirculation. TCD and angiograms are very sensitive for the detection of vasospasm in the large arterial segments but much less accurate when cerebral vasospasm is more distal. Thus, patients may develop ischemic lesions, particularly in deep brain regions, despite having normal or near-normal velocities on TCD and vessel diameters on cerebral angiogram. CT perfusion scans only partially overcome this limitation because their

TABLE 9.1  **Risk Factors for the Development of Delayed Cerebral Ischemia after aSAH**

Extensive clot in subarachnoid cisterns on admission CT scan *

Intraventricular hemorrhage on CT scan within first 24 hours*

Young age

Active smoking

Cocaine use

Poor clinical neurologic examination at onset

* Factors considered in the modified Fisher scale: grade 0, no SAH or IVH; grade 1, thin SAH without IVH; grade 2, thin SAH with IVH; grade 3, thick SAH without IVH; grade 4, thick SAH with IVH.

| Diagnostic modality | Parameter evaluated |
|---|---|
| Catheter angiography | Large vessel spasm |
| Transcranial Doppler | Large vessel spasm (circle of Willis) VMR with $CO_2$ challenge |
| CT angiography | Large vessel spasm |
| CT perfusion | Cerebral perfusion |
| MR angiography | Large vessel spasm |
| MRI with DWI/PWI | Cerebral perfusion and early ischemia |
| SPECT | Cerebral perfusion |
| Jugular oximetry | Regional brain oxygenation |
| Brain tissue O2 | Local brain oxygenation |

VMR, vasomotor reactivity

interpretation in practice relies on side-to-side comparison, which loses value in common cases of diffuse, bilateral cerebral vasospasm. CT perfusion may show hypoperfusion much more clearly in the cortex than in the deep white matter. Since ischemia can occur in the absence of documented vasospasm (either because we do not have the right tools to identify it or because there are mechanisms other than reductions in arterial luminal diameter causing the ischemia) the term "delayed cerebral ischemia" is more appropriate than "symptomatic cerebral vasospasm."

When we suspect a patient is having delayed cerebral ischemia we initiate hemodynamic augmentation therapy. The former approach of the "triple H" (hypervolemia, hypertension, hemodilution) has fallen out of favor for good reasons. Hypervolemia is not sufficient to produce a sustained increase in cerebral blood flow and perfusion. Furthermore, it can impair brain oxygenation and it is the main cause of cardiopulmonary complications in these patients. Hemodilution, if excessive, can compromise oxygen-carrying capacity and result in insufficient brain oxygen delivery. Thus, we rely mostly on inducing hypertension after ensuring a normovolemic state.

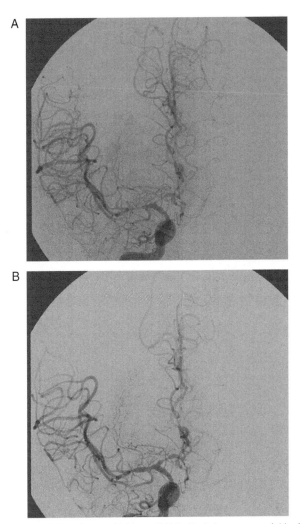

**FIGURE 9.2** A) Cerebral angiogram (right carotid injection) shows severe right middle cerebral artery vasospasm. B) Good angiographic result after treatment with balloon angioplasty.

Most frequently we use phenylephrine or norepinephrine, depending on the initial heart rate and the cardiac status, and we aim to increase the mean arterial pressure by 20–25% as the first step. If symptoms persist, we keep raising the blood pressure, sometimes reaching mean arterial pressures of

140 mmHg. When induced hypertension fails to yield clinical improvement or patients cannot tolerate this medical treatment (e.g., patients with advanced coronary artery disease, heart failure from chronic hypertension, ischemic cardiomyopathy or apical ballooning syndrome), we pursue endovascular therapies, i.e., angioplasty when possible or intra-arterial infusion of a calcium channel blocker.

Our patient was treated with hemodynamic augmentation followed by angioplasty of the right middle cerebral artery (Figure 9.2). Her neurological deficits improved, and she recovered favorably over the subsequent days. Eight weeks later she had returned to work as a teacher.

It is no surprise that "good grade" patients with aSAH may rapidly become "poor grade" patients. The causes are well documented. They just need to be recognized and treated rapidly. Care provided by a dedicated team of neuroscience nurses and skilled physicians with expertise in the management of aSAH is essential to reduce the morbidity of this disease.

---

**KEY POINTS TO REMEMBER REGARDING NEUROLOGICAL WORSENING AFTER SUBARACHNOID HEMORRHAGE**

- The causes of neurological decline in aSAH relate to the time from aneurysm rupture.
- During the first few hours consider rebleeding if the decline is catastrophic and hydrocephalus if the patient drifts into stupor.
- Many patients with aSAH may benefit from a ventriculostomy.
- Cerebral vasospasm typically occurs after the third day from aneurysm rupture. It often presents with subtle changes in cognition and attention before focal deficits are noted. It remains very difficult to confidently diagnose this condition and there are no accurate non-invasive ways to do it.
- TCD, CT perfusion scan, and cerebral angiogram are useful to monitor and document vasospasm, but the diagnosis of delayed cerebral ischemia remains primarily clinical.
- Induced hypertension is the most useful medical treatment to reverse ischemic symptoms. Endovascular therapy is necessary when symptoms are refractory.

## Further Reading

Frontera JA, Fernandez A, Schmidt JM et al. Clinical response to hypertensive hypervolemic therapy and outcome after subarachnoid hemorrhage. *Neurosurgery* 2010; 66:35–41.

Jun P, Ko NU, English JD, Dowd CF, Halbach VV, Higashida RT, Lawton MT, Hetts SW. Endovascular treatment of medically refractory cerebral vasospasm following aneurysmal subarachnoid hemorrhage. *AJNR Am J Neuroradiol* 2010; 31:1911–1916.

Hasan D, Vermeulen M, Wijdicks EFM et al. Management problems in acute hydrocephalus after subarachnoid hemorrhage. *Stroke* 1989; 20:747–753.

Kumar R, Friedman JA. Subarachnoid hemorrhage:the first 24 hours.A surgeon's perspective. *Neurocrit Care* 2011;14:287–290.

Rabinstein AA. Secondary brain injury after aneurysmal subarachnoid hemorrhage: more than vasospasm. *Lancet Neurol* 2011;10:593–595.

Rabinstein AA, Friedman JA, Weigand SD et al. Predictors of cerebral infarction in aneurysmal subarachnoid hemorrhage. *Stroke* 2004; 35:1862–1866.

Rabinstein AA, Lanzino G, Wijdicks EFM. Multidisciplinary management and emerging therapeutic strategies in aneurysmal subarachnoid haemorrhage. *Lancet Neurol* 2010; 9:504–519.

Rabinstein AA, Wijdicks EFM. Cerebral vasospasm in subarachnoid hemorrhage. *Curr Treat Options Neurol* 2005; 7:99–107.

# Options in Acute Spinal Cord Compression

A 90-year-old male in perfect condition and no major medical history presents with 3-week onset of dull back pain. The pain is nagging, but not shooting and with no tingling or electrical shock-like sensations. He denies any sensory symptoms or urinary retention. His wife tells us that he had noted some leg weakness and had frequent falls. When specifically asked, she mentions that he has had a 20-pound weight loss. His neurologic examination reveals he is able to walk, but he has proximal leg muscle weakness (MRC 4/5). No sensory level is found. Tendon reflexes are subclonus. There is percussion pain at the thoracic spine level. CT and MRI shows destructive lesions in the left superior pubic ramus and multiple other lesions in the spine. The largest lesion is at T7 involving the posterior body pedicle with epidural extension and spinal cord displacement (Figure 10.1). A PSA level is over 400 ng/ml. He has a fair amount of pain, but believes his leg weakness is not worsening. His wife is not so sure.

**What do you do now?**

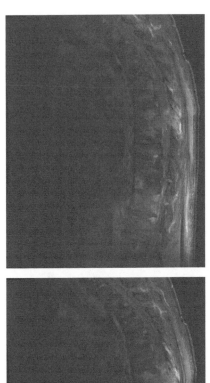

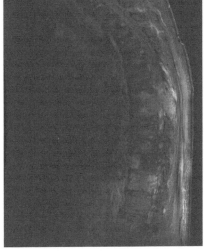

**FIGURE 10.1** Large T7 lesion compressing the cord.

Cancer can take a significant and profound turn for the worse with spinal cord compression. Spinal cord compression may be a presenting symptom of metastatic disease, as it is in our patient example. Such a serious presentation requires a careful assessment of treatment options and there are a few.

Decisions to go ahead with surgical decompression are generally guided by the oncological prognosis—this is not as straightforward as it may seem—and the prediction of ambulation in a patient who has pretreatment motor function. What is mostly true is that a patient who can walk at the time of the intervention will continue to walk, and patients who have developed motor deficits slowly may have a better outcome than patients with more rapid onset. Life expectancy prediction in general has been difficult, but scoring systems have been devised. One example is the Tokuhashi score (Table 10.1). There are several elements that take life expectancy into account and in this scoring system, the primary site of the neoplasm and the neurologic deficit are the most important elements to predict survival.

In our patient the first priority is an assessment of the degree of metastatic epidural compression of the spinal cord. The potential instability of the spine is unquestionably severe.

There are several ways to approach this clinical problem medically and surgically (Table 10.2). Corticosteroids are administered immediately in all patients. There is little certainty whether a high-dose dexamethasone (96 mg per day) or moderate dose (16 mg per day) should be used. Most physicians would prefer an aggressive approach in patients who have had rapid progressive motor symptoms and use a high dose.

The next priority is to determine whether the patient is a surgical candidate. In patients with pain only, stable neurologic findings and a radiosensitive tumor, radiotherapy is the first option. Criteria that have been used to favor an operative management include rapid progression of motor deficit, instability of the spine on MRI scan, medically intractable pain, and incomplete neurologic injury. Some algorithms also include complete sensory and motor paraplegia over 24 hours as a reason to proceed with surgery. However, external-beam radiotherapy is used in most patients, and this requires a total of 30 GY in 10 fractions. Radiotherapy is not considered in radioresistant tumors, such as renal cell carcinoma. If the tumor is not radiosensitive,

| Parameter | Score |
|---|---|
| General Condition | |
| Poor | 0 |
| Moderate | 1 |
| Good | 2 |
| No. of extraspinal metastases | |
| >3 | 0 |
| 1-2 | 1 |
| 0 | 2 |
| No. of vertebral body metastases | |
| >3 | 0 |
| 2 | 1 |
| 1 | 2 |
| Metastases to the major internal organs | |
| Nonremovable | 0 |
| Removable | 1 |
| None | 2 |
| Primary site of cancer | |
| Lung, stomach, bladder, bone | 0 |
| Esophagus, pancreas, liver, gallbladder, unidentified | 1 |
| Others | 2 |
| Kidney, uterus | 3 |
| Rectum | 4 |
| Thyroid, breast, prostate, carcinoid | 5 |

(*Continues*)

TABLE 10.1  **(Cont'd.)**

| Parameter | Score |
|---|---|
| Palsy or myelopathy | |
| Complete | 0 |
| Incomplete | 1 |
| None | 2 |

The information in this table is based on Tokuhashi et al. The lower the score, the worse the prognosis. Those patients scoring from 0 to 8 have a prognosis of less than 6 months to live; a score of 9–11, between 6 and 12 months; and a score of 12 to 15, more than a year.

vertebroplasty or kyphoplasty with or without open stabilization surgery is an option.

Pain treatment is essential not only before but also during and after radiotherapy. There are many options for adequate pain management. A typical approach is using transdermal patches of fentanyl that can be changed every three to four days, oxycodone 10 to 20 mg every two hours as needed, or hydromorphone 4 mg every four hours. This generally provides good pain palliation. For patients with significant neuropathic pain—that may come later—gabapentin 100 mg twice a day and 300 mg at bedtime is a good starting dose; the medication should be then titrated to

TABLE 10.2  **Initial Treatment Options in Acute Spinal Cord Compression from Cancer**

Assess surgical options
    Tokuhashi score
    Good surgical candidate?
    Instability?

Assess radiotherapy option
    Radiosensitive?
    Degree of spinal cord compression?

Assess options to minimize effect of tumor
    Corticosteroids
    Opioids
    Bisphosphonates
    Chemotherapy

between 1,800 and 3,600 mg per day. Bone pain adjuvants are necessary as well, and this includes zoledronic acid 4 mg intravenously every three to four weeks or pamidronate 90 mg intravenously every three to four weeks. Most patients would need bladder catheterization and mostly can learn self-catheterization. Bowel regimen medication is also provided with bisacodyl or glycerin suppository daily, and docusate plus senna.

So what were the decisions in our patient? His Tokuhashi revised score was 10, thus predicting 6 to 12 months of life expectancy. The patient underwent an orchidectomy that resulted in a good response based on his PSA. He was reluctant to undergo surgery and favored radiotherapy first. He was planned to undergo two to five radiation cycles, but unfortunately after three radiation therapies, he fairly rapidly became paraplegic. This resulted in immediate decompressive surgery, but the paraplegia persisted. Despite this motor deficit he remained relatively functional and lived for another 4 years.

This case illustrates well how difficult it is to choose radiotherapy over surgery. In this patient, the decision to postpone surgery seemed justified due to his advanced age and absence of any major neurologic deficit. The sudden appearance of paraplegia may have had a vascular cause, as ischemic myelopathy is not uncommon in these cases. It is uncertain whether this could have been prevented with earlier epidural decompression. Life expectancy prediction after epidural spine compression is difficult and remains a gross estimation. This is particularly the case in patients with metastatic prostate cancer when there is good response to castration, since they may have an extended period of time with reasonable quality of life.

---

**KEY POINTS TO REMEMBER REGARDING OPTIONS IN ACUTE SPINAL CORD COMPRESSION**

- Outcome after epidural cord compression is dependent on the type of tumor, radiosensitivity, rapidity of progression of neurologic symptoms, and instability of the spine.
- Aggressive surgical management is not indicated if there is pain only and no major neurologic deficit.
- Aggressive pain management with opioids and corticosteroids may provide adequate palliation.

- Which treatment modality is best for the patient is determined based on severity and acuity of the neurologic deficit, nature of the tumor, instability of the spine, and general performance status and life expectancy of the patient.

### Further Reading

Abrahm JL, Banffy MB, Harris MB. Spinal cord compression in patients with advanced metastatic cancer. *JAMA* 2008; 299:937-946.

Cole JS, Patchell RA. Metastatic epidural spinal cord compression. *Lancet Neurol* 2008; 7:459-466.

Graber JJ, Nolan CP. Myelopathies in patients with cancer. *Arch Neurol* 2010; 67:298-304.

Prasad D, Schiff D. Malignant spinal-cord compression. *Lancet Oncol* 2005; 6:15-24.

Quraishi NA, Gokaslan ZL, Boriani S. The surgical management of metastatic epidural compression of the spinal cord. *J Bone Surg Br.* 2010; 92-B:1054-1060.

Tokuhashi Y, Matsuaki H, Oda H et al. A revised scoring system for preoperative evaluation of metastatic spine tumor prognosis. *Spine* 2005; 30:2186-2191.

# Choices in Refractory Status Epilepticus

A 42-year-old woman with history of epilepsy was brought to our emergency department after having three witnessed generalized tonic-clonic seizures. Her epilepsy was a result of prior traumatic head injury. Recently the dose of valproic acid had been reduced. The paramedics decided to intubate her prior to transportation due to concerns about the patency of her airway. We are called into the emergency department to evaluate the patient, when she has another generalized tonic-clonic seizure upon our arrival. The seizure lasts 90 seconds and the patient remains unconscious after its conclusion. Her husband informs us that she has not been alert since the first seizure happened. She is intubated and mechanically ventilated with good oxygenation, afebrile, and mildly tachycardic and hypertensive. She has no neck stiffness and no lateralizing signs on motor examination. We lift her eyelids and notice nystagmus-like movements of her eyes.

**What do you do now?**

Successful treatment of status epilepticus (SE) begins with the recognition that it is a neurological emergency. If you don't treat it early, SE becomes more refractory over time. This is due to pharmacoresistance and alteration in the GABA receptor sensitivity and availability to agonists, such as benzodiazepines. The longer it lasts the higher the risk of complications, including permanent neuronal damage and dropout.

The questions we should ask ourselves are: First, how do you recognize refractory SE? In patients with continuous generalized convulsions the diagnosis of SE is self-evident (though it still requires differentiation from psychogenic pseudo-SE). But, all too often, there seems to be reluctance to diagnose SE in patients with rapidly repetitive seizures. These patients must be treated for SE if they do not recover full alertness between seizures. The diagnosis is also missed too frequently when the clinical manifestations are subtle (for instance in cases of complex partial SE) and when patients are comatose (in whom the only clinical manifestation, if any, may be nystagmoid eye movements or minimal flickering of a finger or a toe). Generalized convulsive SE becomes nonconvulsive over time, and EEG recording is often needed to find a close correlation between subtle movements and ictal discharges.

Second, how do you treat SE when it becomes refractory? Even the suspicion of SE means you must start antiepileptic treatment immediately. Benzodiazepines are the first-line therapy—intravenous lorazepam being the preferred choice because of its rapid onset of action and longer duration of antiepileptic effect—and should be given while emergently assessing airway patency, adequacy of ventilation and oxygenation, and circulatory status. In all cases a capillary glucose level should be measured to exclude hypoglycemia. Blood should be drawn for measurement of serum electrolytes, lactic acid, creatine kinase, complete cell count, and arterial gases. If seizures stop and the patient wakes up, further progression is not likely. But if the seizures do not stop you need to move to the next line of therapy (fosphenytoin or valproic acid) without delay. In fact, treatment of SE is best optimized by following a clear protocol progressing from one line of therapy to the next until seizures stop. The dose should be adequate, and failure to prescribe the right dose is a common error. Always check if the patient has received an appropriate dose of each drug (e.g., lorazepam 0.1 mg/kg, phosphenytoin 20 mg/kg or higher, valproic acid 30 mg/kg or higher) before concluding it failed. Our current treatment protocol is shown in Figure 11.1.

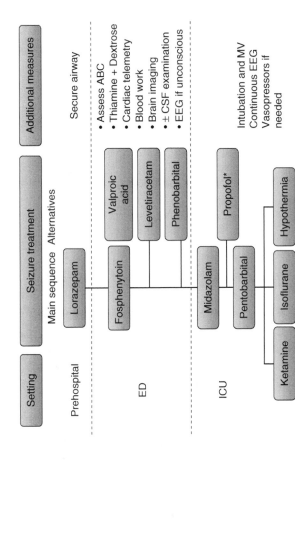

**FIGURE 11.1** Algorithm for the management of status epilepticus. ABC, airway, breathing, circulation; CSF, cerebrospinal fluid; ED, emergency department; EEG, electroencephalography; ICU, intensive care unit; MV, mechanical ventilation.

*The risk of propofol infusion syndrome is substantial and this complication may be fatal.

SE should be considered refractory after failure of two antiepileptic agents. In our practice, the diagnosis of refractory generalized SE means we will need to start a continuous infusion of an anesthetic agent. This decision demands endotracheal intubation for mechanical ventilation and continuous electroencephalographic (EEG) monitoring. There are some exceptions to this rule. In cases of complex partial status epilepticus we try one or two more anticonvulsants before using anesthetics because in these patients there is less evidence that uncontrolled complex partial seizures can produce irreversible brain damage, at least in the short term. For the same reasons, in patients with epilepsia partialis continua we try to avoid intubation and potent anesthetic drugs.

Among anesthetic agents we favor midazolam because of its better safety profile (Table 11.1). Midazolam can be effective in aborting status epilepticus when used in high doses. We start with a bolus of 0.2 mg per kilogram of body weight and an infusion of 0.2 mg/kg/hr. However, we rapidly increase the infusion dose until we achieve suppression of the seizures and have reached doses as high as 5 mg/kg/hr in the most recalcitrant cases. Even these very high doses are well tolerated by most patients, although support with vasopressor drugs may be needed. Tachyphylaxis develops quickly with benzodiazepines in general and midazolam in particular. This phenomenon may demand using even higher doses if the infusion needs to be maintained over time.

Propofol is a very effective antiepileptic anesthetic, but we have found it unsafe in the doses necessary to control refractory SE (often higher than 100 micrograms per kg per minute). The main risk is the development of propofol infusion syndrome. This syndrome –albeit rare– is manifested by lactic acidosis, rhabdomyolysis, myocardial depression, and, when most severe, cardiovascular collapse and cardiac arrest. In our experience, even careful monitoring of metabolic changes (serial lactic acid, arterial blood gases, and creatine kinase levels) may fail to recognize the beginning of a fatal form of this complication. Therefore, we rarely use propofol for the treatment of SE and when we do we strictly avoid infusing large doses. More than 80 µg/kg per minute or 3 mg/kg per hour for longer than 48 hours should be avoided.

Continuous infusion of barbiturates, such as pentobarbital, is very effective in aborting SE. Unfortunately, adverse side effects are many and often severe. Hypotension is ubiquitous and requires vasopressors.

TABLE 11.1 **Doses and Side Effects of Therapeutic Options for Refractory Status Epilepticus**

| Drug | Dose | Infusion rate | Major side effects |
|---|---|---|---|
| Lorazepam | 0.1 mg/kg | 2 mg/min | Sedation<br>Respiratory depression |
| Diazepam | 0.2 mg/kg | 5 mg/min | Sedation<br>Respiratory depression |
| Fosphenytoin | 20 mg/kg | 150 mg/min | Hypotension<br>Cardiac arrhythmia |
| Valproic acid | 25-45 mg/kg | Up to 6 mg/kg/min | Severe encephalopathy if high ammonia or mitochondrial disorder |
| Levetiracetam | 20-40 mg/kg | Over 5-15 min | Mild sedation |
| Phenobarbital | 15-20 mg/kg | 100 mg/min | Hypotension<br>Respiratory depression |
| Midazolam | 0.2 mg/kg | 0.2 to 5 mg/kg/hr* | Sedation<br>Hypotension<br>Respiratory depression |
| Propofol | 2 mg/kg | 40 to 200 mcg/kg/min | Sedation<br>Hypotension<br>Respiratory depression<br>Propofol infusion syndrome** |
| Pentobarbital | 5-10 mg/kg | 1-5 mg/kg/hr | Prolonged sedation<br>Hypotension<br>Respiratory depression<br>Myocardial depression<br>Infections (pneumonia)<br>Liver dysfunction<br>Ileus<br>Early skin breakdown<br>Drug interactions |

*Usual doses are between 0.2 and 5 mg/kg/hr, but much higher rates of infusion are needed (and can be tolerated) in selected cases.

**Life-threatening risk with prolonged infusion of high doses of the drug; contraindicated in children.

Infections, especially pneumonia, ileus, and liver toxicity occur in the majority of patients treated with a barbiturate drip for more than 2 days. Consequently, we tend to reserve this option for those patients who fail to be controlled with midazolam.

There are other alternatives we have tried with variable success in our most challenging cases. We have not been impressed by the usefulness of lidocaine and ketamine, but others have noticed good results using high doses of ketamine. We have found isoflurane to be the only effective rescue therapy in patients who had become dependent on very high doses of pentobarbital. Our enthusiasm for isoflurane has been tempered, however, by the appearance of marked brain and brainstem abnormalities on the MRI scans in two of our isoflurane-treated patients suggesting a neurotoxic effect.

Induced hypothermia can also be helpful in SE. Our experience with hypothermia for this indication is still limited, but our initial results have been encouraging. Finally, in some cases the seizures can only be controlled by treating the underlying cause that provoked them. Searching for treatable forms of encephalitis, brain lesions amenable to resection, and some specific systemic illnesses (for instance thrombotic thrombocytopenic purpura) is equally important. Last-resort measures have included ketogenic diet or electroconvulsive therapy. How electroconvulsive therapy works is not known and may be simply through a "rebooting" phenomenon. In the worst cases, one must accept at some point that the status epilepticus is untreatably refractory; in these rare instances the status eventually "burns out" at the expense of rapid brain loss which can be documented by the accelerated atrophy on serial neuroimaging.

Back to our patient. After another seizure in the emergency department she was treated with 0.1 mg/kg of intravenous lorazepam. The abnormal eye movements only resolved for a few minutes but then recurred. Because valproate discontinuation likely triggered the seizures, she was loaded with valproic acid (15 mg/kg while awaiting the serum level) and then transferred her to our neurosciences intensive care unit. Emergency EEG showed continuous epileptiform activity. After a bolus of 0.2 mg/kg, midazolam infusion was initiated in the ICU at a rate of 0.2 mg/kg/hr and then titrated until the electrographic seizures abated (infusion rate reached 0.5 mg/kg/hr). We then adjusted the dose of valproic acid according to the serum level, which was subtherapeutic. Within the following 24 hours we were able to wean off the infusion of midazolam. The patient awoke and could be extubated without problems.

Treatment of refractory status epilepticus may be summarized as follows: treat aggressively and early and neurologists should pack a hard punch, protect and support the patient, and try to find a treatable cause. Even when prolonged anesthetic treatment is needed, outcome can still be favorable in young patients if there is no MRI evidence of permanent brain damage.

---

**KEY POINTS TO REMEMBER REGARDING CHOICES IN REFRACTORY STATUS EPILEPTICUS**

- Status epilepticus is a neurological emergency.
- Seizures become more resistant to antiepileptics over time, and prolonged status epilepticus can produce irreversible brain damage.
- It is best to use a treatment protocol and to decisively progress from step to step.
- Make sure the right drugs and the right doses are being used.
- If two anticonvulsants fail, consider intubating the patient, use continuous electroencephalographic monitoring, and starting a continuous infusion of an anesthetic agent.
- Among anesthetics, midazolam provides the best balance between safety and effectiveness. Propofol and pentobarbital are also very effective, but their use is associated with a greater risk of severe- and even fatal medical complications.
- Inhaled gases, such as isoflurane, and moderate hypothermia are valuable therapeutic alternatives in recalcitrant cases.

---

**Further Reading**

Chen JW, Wasterlain CG. Status epilepticus: pathophysiology and management in adults. *Lancet Neurol* 2006; 5:246-256.

Cooper AD, Britton JW, Rabinstein AA. Functional and cognitive outcome in prolonged refractory status epilepticus. *Arch Neurol* 2009; 66:1505-1509.

Fugate JE, Burns JD, Wijdicks EF, Warner DO, Jankowski CJ, Rabinstein AA. Prolonged high-dose isoflurane for refractory status epilepticus: is it safe? *Anesth Analg* 2010; 111:1520-1524.

Iyer VN, Hoel R, Rabinstein AA. Propofol infusion syndrome in patients with refractory status epilepticus: an 11-year clinical experience. *Crit Care Med* 2009; 37:3024–3030.

Mayer SA, Claassen J, Lokin J, Mendelsohn F, Dennis LJ, Fitzsimmons BF. Refractory status epilepticus: frequency, risk factors, and impact on outcome. *Arch Neurol* 2002; 59:205–210.

Meierkord H, Boon P, Engelsen B, Göcke K, Shorvon S, Tinuper P, Holtkamp M; European Federation of Neurological Societies. EFNS guideline on the management of status epilepticus in adults. *Eur J Neurol* 2010; 17:348–355.

Rabinstein AA. Management of status epilepticus in adults. *Neurol Clin* 2010; 28:853–862.

Shorvon S. The treatment of status epilepticus. *Curr Opin Neurol.* 2011; 24:165–170.

A 64-year-old man with history of smoking was admitted after having recurrent episodes of loss of consciousness over the last 2 days. For the previous 3-4 weeks he had been having more problems with concentration and worsening gait balance. He also noticed that he was not seeing well on the right side and had difficulties with left hand movements. Upon evaluation in our emergency department he was fully awake but his answers were slow. He had a right visual field deficit and left-sided ataxia. A CT scan showed masses in the left cerebellar hemisphere and the left parietooccipital region surrounded by fairly extensive edema. He was started on dexamethasone. Anticipating decline despite administration of corticosteroids and the possibility of an urgent neurosurgical debulking, he was admitted to our NICU for close observation. Twelve hours after arrival his condition declined. On examination he is difficult to awaken and has developed left facial and abducens nerve palsies.

**What do you do now?**

Malignancies may present anywhere in the brain and cause rapid decline even before the pathology is known. Patients with a primary malignant brain tumor may worsen quickly from growth of the tumor size, but the most common causes for decline are increasing edema and new hemorrhage (Table 12.1). The more aggressive the tumor, the higher is the likelihood of these two complications. Highly malignant tumors secrete angiogenic factors, which promote the rapid formation of intratumoral vessels. The lack of efficient tight junctions in these vessels produces a disruption of the blood brain barrier, which results in the formation of vasogenic edema. These vessels are also immature and thus fragile and prone to rupture.

Patients with malignant brain tumors may also deteriorate as a result of exacerbating factors that disturb ongoing compensatory mechanisms. For instance, seizures can produce hypoventilation and hypercapnia from a reduced respiratory drive, which in turn can lead to increased cerebral blood volume and worsening tissue shift in patients with exhausted intracranial compliance. Incremental administration of opiates for excruciating headaches can have similar consequences. Severe hyponatremia, sometimes related to inadequate secretion of antidiuretic hormone, as a paraneoplastic disorder or due to hydrocephalus, can worsen cerebral edema. Radiation therapy, although useful for the reduction of mass effect in the longer term, is characteristically associated with worsening inflammatory edema in the early phase.

So what options do we have for our patient? Corticosteroids are very useful for the treatment of peritumoral vasogenic edema and often high

TABLE 12.1  **Causes of Neurological Deterioration in Patients with Malignant Brain Tumors**

Worsening of vasogenic peritumoral edema*

Intratumoral hemorrhage*

Seizures with prolonged recovery of aphasia or hemiparesis

Obstructive hydrocephalus

Venous infarction from extension of the tumor to the dural sinus

Arterial infarction from vessel invasion or compression by the tumor

*By far the two most common

doses are necessary. We adjust the dose depending on the severity of the edema. In patients with preserved alertness and no substantial brain tissue shift the usual dose of 10 mg of dexamethasone may suffice. However, we administer intravenous bolus doses of 20–100 mg in severe and extreme cases. Maintenance doses then range from 4 to 10 mg every 4 to 6 hours. When using high-dose steroids it is essential to minimize the risks and to initiate preventive measures (Table 12.2). Even if administered early, intravenous dexamethasone may take hours to reach its maximum effect and patients may deteriorate before that time. Other anti-edema medical treatments (mannitol or hypertonic saline) only have a role in emergency situations and often are used as a bridge towards surgery.

Surgical treatment is the most effective. If complete resection is not possible, debulking should be considered. Patients who present with rapid clinical worsening and signs of brainstem displacement, those with large

TABLE 12.2 **Short-Term Side Effects and Preventive Measures Related to High-Dose Glucocorticosteroids**

| Side effect | Preventive measure |
| --- | --- |
| Hyperglycemia | Frequent glucose monitoring Insulin scale or continuous infusion |
| Increased susceptibility to infections (especially by *Pneumocystis jiroveci*) | Double-strength trimetroprim sulfamethoxazole 3 times per week |
| Psychosis | Antidopaminergics |
| Mood swings | Mood stabilizers (e.g., valproic acid) |
| Peptic ulcers* | H2 blockers or proton pump inhibitors |
| High blood pressure | Monitoring and treatment as necessary |
| Myopathy | Minimize immobilization |
| Hypokalemia | Potassium monitoring and replacement |

*Risk may only be increased with high doses, when there is severe stress, and after recent use of nonsteroidal anti-inflammatory agents.

intratumoral hemorrhages, and those failing increasing doses of glucocorticosteroids necessitate urgent surgery. Often the decision to operate will have to be made without knowing the primary pathology and thus the prognosis. Biopsies should be generally discouraged in patients with large masses and no space to expand. Even minor postoperative bleeding—a relatively frequent occurrence- can put patients at considerable further risk if the mass effect is not reduced during surgery. As illustrated by our case, cerebellar masses require surgery more often than supratentorial ones. Occasionally, the acute neurological decline may be due to superimposed obstructive hydrocephalus, and in these cases ventricular drainage can be a minimally invasive temporary solution.

Whether patients with known malignant primary brain tumors need urgent or emergent surgery is a complex decision. The previous functional status of the patient, his or her previously stated wishes, the possibility of effective future tumor treatment, and, most important, the potential for recovery of quality of life after surgery have to be carefully considered. The major ethical question in some patients reaching this stage is whether a neurosurgical procedure is justified in a situation that may be hopeless and in which surgery may afford only minimal gain in survival with poor quality of life. Some families are unable to decide, others may have a better perspective and may turn to palliative care.

Our patient had been given 20 mg of dexamethasone and 2,000 mg of levetiracetam (for suspected previous seizures) in the emergency department. When he worsened in the ICU we gave 20 mg more of dexamethasone along with 1 g/kg of 20% mannitol. A repeat CT scan—showed that he had developed obstructive hydrocephalus from aqueductal compression. He underwent urgent surgery for excision of the cerebellar mass (Figure 12.1.) His hydrocephalus resolved and his neurological condition improved. He continued receiving dexamethasone 6 mg every 6 hours with subsequent taper. His CT scan of the chest showed a nodular mass. Lung biopsy and brain pathology showed non–small cell carcinoma. He underwent further treatment and had a good functional status 6 months later.

All patients with a neurosurgical procedure for metastasis from a highly malignant tumor or recurrent brain malignancy will succumb in a short time period. Yet, after aggressive treatment of the brain mass, the quality of life during most of that time can be quite acceptable in some patients.

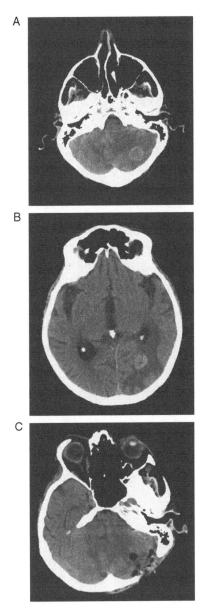

**FIGURE 12.1**  A) Head CT scan showing a left cerebellar mass with associated edema producing effacement of the 4th ventricle. B) At a higher level, a second mass is seen in the left parietooccipital area. Note the dilatation of the third ventricle. C) After surgical excision of the cerebellar mass, the CT scan shows persistent edema with mass effect but less prominent than before and reappearance of a visible 4th ventricle.

- Acute neurological decline from brain metastasis or malignant brain tumor is most frequently due to worsening vasogenic edema or hemorrhage.
- Precipitating causes (such as seizures, hypoventilation, and hyponatremia) need to be recognized and treated without delay.
- Glucocorticosteroids are the best medical treatment for vasogenic edema.
- Surgical treatment (tumor removal or debulking) becomes urgent or emergent in rapidly deteriorating patients, presence of a large hemorrhage, and patients refractory to medical treatments. When offering surgery as a life-saving intervention, the future prognosis and wishes of the patient need to be discussed in detail.

**Further Reading**

Linskey ME, Andrews DW, Asher AL, Burri SH, Kondziolka D, Robinson PD, Ammirati M, Cobbs CS, Gaspar LE, Loeffler JS, McDermott M, Mehta MP, Mikkelsen T, Olson JJ, Paleologos NA, Patchell RA, Ryken TC, Kalkanis SN. The role of stereotactic radiosurgery in the management of patients with newly diagnosed brain metastases: a systematic review and evidence-based clinical practice guideline. *J Neurooncol* 2010; 96:45-68.

Qureshi AI, Geocadin RG, Suarez JI et al. Long-term outcome after medical reversal of transtentorial herniation in patients with supratentorial mass lesions. *Crit Care Med* 2000; 28:1556-1564.

Ranjan T, Abrey LE. Current management of metastatic brain disease. *Neurotherapeutics.* 2009;6:598-603.

Ryken TC, McDermott M, Robinson PD et al. The role of steroids in the management of brain metastases: a systematic review and evidence-based clinical practice guideline. *J Neurooncol* 2010; 96:103-114.

Silbergeld DL, Rostomily RC, Alvord EC Jr. The cause of death in patients with glioblastoma is multifactorial: clinical factors and autopsy findings in 117 cases of supratentorial glioblastoma in adults. *J Neurooncol* 1991; 10:179-185.

Stiver SI. Angiogenesis and its role in the behavior of astrocytic brain tumors. *Front Biosci* 2004; 9:3105-3123.

Wen PY, Schiff D, Kesari S, Drappatz J, Gigas DC, Doherty L. Medical management of patients with brain tumors. *J Neurooncol* 2006; 80:313-332.

# 13 Hypothermia After Cardiopulmonary Resuscitation

A 61-year-old woman slumped down with rattling breathing and rapidly developing cyanosis. A bystander performed cardiopulmonary resuscitation, but the EMS arrived quickly and documented ventricular fibrillation. Several shocks were needed to restore circulation. The patient remained comatose and was intubated. External ice packs and iced saline was used during transportation, and after arrival to the intensive care unit, the patient was cooled to 33°C using an external cooling device. An EEG showed suppressed activity but changed to epileptiform discharges during rewarming. Somatosensory-evoked potentials showed absent $N_{20}$ response on the right side. Serum neuron specific enolase is 55 ng/mL. The patient still requires substantial amount of vasopressors and inotropes for a failing heart. Neurologic examination two days after rewarming reveals no eye opening to pain, no motor response to pain, intact pupil responses to light, normal corneal reflexes, intact grimacing, and cough response to suctioning. The family wants to know what to expect, as does the cardiologist.

*What do you do now?*

Neurologists seem to be the arbiters of gloomy events in coronary care units, but that may change in the era of therapeutic hypothermia. The truth is that even when comatose patients are cooled immediately after cardiopulmonary resuscitation (CPR), the chance of survival is still about 50/50, and many patients die within a week from withdrawal of support. Hypothermia is now considered standard of care for patients with out-of-hospital arrest from ventricular fibrillation, and a protocol is shown in Table 13.1. Hypothermia protocols—as expected—vary considerably across centers, and this also applies to utilization. Selection of patients also varies with an increasing number of centers, including patients with asystole and in-hospital arrest. Yet, there is no evidence that therapeutic hypothermia is effective under these circumstances. More and more hospitals are set up to provide therapeutic hypothermia, but neurologists currently may see just about equal numbers of patients with or without hypothermia treatment.

Poor predictors of outcome at the time of resuscitation have been identified and the cardiac rhythm causing circulatory arrest is a major determinant of outcome. Outcome of patients with a "nonshockable" rhythm (asystole, pulseless electrical activity) is poor, but rapid defibrillation in other rhythms (ventricular fibrillation, ventricular tachycardia) may be successful, resulting in rapid awakening of the patient and even the probability of intact neurologic function.

**TABLE 13.1  Hypothermia Protocol in Comatose Survivors after Cardiopulmonary Resuscitation**

1.5 liter of refrigerated (4-6 °C) saline in 30-60 minutes

Operate cooling device to 33 °C

Monitor bladder temperature

Sedate patient before paralysis

Sedate with Midazolam 0.3 mg/kg/hr IV and Fentanyl 0.1 mcg/kg/hr IV

Paralyze (to prevent shivering) with Atracurium 0.2 mg/kg

Normalize serum magnesium and potassium values

Normalize serum glucose values

Monitor electrolytes, WBC, and platelets

Monitor EEG/video during rewarming and for 24 hours (if available)

The clinical picture of postcardiac resuscitation syndrome is concerning. Patients may have a major myocardial dysfunction (which may be reversible), a systemic ischemic-reperfusion syndrome with intravascular volume depletion, for a full-blown acute coronary syndrome requiring reperfusion strategies. More invasive treatments such as extracorporeal membrane oxygenation may be necessary in some cases. A profound kidney and liver injury may be present. The response to treatment of these complications plays an important role in planning the level of care.

The neurological examination is focused on motor response, presence of spontaneous eye movements, appearance of myoclonus or seizures and whether there has been brainstem injury resulting in changes in key brainstem reflexes. The immediate presence of localizing motor responses is the best evidence that the duration of ischemia to the brain has been brief. Long duration of circulatory arrest results in a more profound insult and may be apparent by the documentation of abnormal extensor or flexor response or no response to a noxious stimulus in the arms and legs. Motor response after CPR, however, has never been a very reliable predictor of outcome even before the wide application of induced hypothermia. Patients with withdrawal responses to pain may not wake up or may regain only minimal consciousness. Of even greater concern is myoclonic status epilepticus. Myoclonus involves the face, limbs, and axial muscles. These brief jerks are spontaneous and in the first hours after CPR may be unrelenting and forceful. It may make the patient move in the bed and cause considerable upset to family members.

Brainstem reflexes are typically normal because the brainstem is often spared from anoxic-ischemic injury. Absent brainstem reflexes may occur after prolonged periods of resuscitation or in resuscitation of trauma patients with substantial blood loss. Fixed and dilated pupils are more frequently associated with asystole than with ventricular fibrillation and that may simply be a reflection of more prolonged anoxic- ischemic brain injury. Fixed and dilated pupils throughout the resuscitation procedure usually indicate a poor chance of success. Successful cardiac resuscitation with good neurologic recovery more often occurs in patients with persistently contracted and reactive pupils from the onset.

Prognostic factors for poor neurologic outcome have been identified in a recent evidence-based guideline from the American Academy of Neurology

**TABLE 13.2** **Poor Outcome Anticipated**

| | |
|---|---|
| 0-24 hours | Myoclonus status epilepticus |
| 24-72 hours | SSEP: absent cortical ($N_{20}$) responses |
| 24-72 hours | Serum NSE > 33 ug/L* |
| > 72 hours | Absent pupil or corneal reflexes<br>Extensor motor responses<br>Absent motor responses* |

* These findings are not as reliable after therapeutic hypothermia

(Table 13.2). Several of these factors may be difficult to reliably assess due to use of sedative and analgesic agents needed with therapeutic hypothermia, and particularly the reliability of the motor response is currently questioned. Moreover the prognostic value of a single sample of serum neuron specific enolase (NSE) is very uncertain (serial measurements showing an increase may have more value, but this remains to be proven). Failure to awaken several days after cardiopulmonary resuscitation may prompt MR imaging, but studies on its prognostic importance are yet not definitive. However, finding diffuse laminar cortical necrosis in an unchanged comatose patient likely predicts a poor outcome (nursing home and major functional disability).

So how do we approach this patient? First, there is a renewed concern that patients in therapeutic hypothermia—who are also paralyzed—may be actively seizing, and failure to treat seizures may result in worse outcome. No evidence has yet been presented that aggressive management of seizures (and in particular subclinical status epilepticus) may impact outcome. Generalized epileptiform discharges or overt epileptic seizures (without clinical accompaniment of myoclonus status epilepticus) may occur and can be treated with additional increasing doses of midazolam. However, patients with EEG patterns of status epilepticus, burst suppression, or generalized suppression with no reactivity remain comatose despite aggressive antiepileptic drug administration. It is far more likely these EEG patterns reflect severe anoxic-ischemic injury rather than a treatable condition. The value of aggressive treatment of these "malignant" EEG patterns is thus very doubtful and there has not been published evidence to the contrary.

Second, we usually proceed with summarizing clinical signs and laboratory data that are inarguably linked to poor prognosis in a comatose patient. In our patient we did not find myoclonus status epilepticus or loss or pupil and cornea reflexes, SSEP showed a preserved cortical ($N_{20}$) response on one side, and only the NSE was elevated (an uncertain finding in patients treated with hypothermia). Thus, in our patient's example, we were unable to prognosticate with certainty, and continued support was warranted. The patient gradually awakened but remained in a severely disabled state requiring nursing home placement. This case illustrates the current limitations of early prognostication in comatose patients treated with therapeutic hypothermia after cardiac resuscitation. The whole notion of being able to tell early on who is going to do well and who is not remains a challenge for the neurologist with only a few clinical cues to go by. We may know who is going to do poorly but we have difficulty predicting who is going to regain independence and recover full use of intellectual capabilities.

## KEY POINTS TO REMEMBER REGARDING HYPOTHERMIA AFTER CARDIOPULMONARY RESUSCITATION

- Certain clinical and laboratory findings are helpful in prognostication. Poor prognosis can be expected in patients with absence of pupillary light responses, corneal reflexes, and an extensor or absent motor response, or myoclonus status epilepticus.
- Documented seizures on EEG may need treatment, but the value of aggressive antiepileptic treatment is uncertain.
- The confounding effects of sedative drugs during hypothermia needs careful judgment.

Further Reading

Chamorro C, Borrallo JM, Romera MA, et al. Anesthesia and analgesia protocol during therapeutic hypothermia after cardiac arrest: a systemic review. *Anesth Analg* 2010;110:1328-1335.

Dumas F, Grimaldi D, Zuber B, et al. Is hypothermia after cardiac arrest effective in both shockable and nonshockable patients?: insights from a large registry. *Circulation*. 2011;123:877-886.

Fugate JE, Wijdicks EFM, Mandrekar J, Claassen DO, Manno EM, White RD, Bell MR, Rabinstein AA. Predictors of neurologic outcome in hypothermia after cardiac arrest. *Ann Neurol* 2010; 68:907-914.

Fugate JE, Wijdicks EFM, White R,Rabinstein AA. Does therapeutic hypothermia affect time to awakening in survivors of cardiopulmonary arrest? *Neurology* 2011, in press

Neumar RW, Nolan JP, Adrie C, Aibiki M, Berg RA, Bottiger BW, Callaway C, Clark RS et al. Post-cardiac arrest syndrome: epidemiology, pathophysiology, treatment, and prognostication. *Int Emerg Nurs* 2010;18:8-28.

Walters JH, Morley PT, Nolan JP. The role of hypothermia in post-cardiac arrest patients with return of spontaneous circulation: a systematic review, *Resuscitation* 2011; 82: 508-516.

Wijdicks EFM, Hijdra A, Young GB, Bassetti CL, Wiebe S; Quality Standards Subcommittee of the American Academy of Neurology. Practice parameter: prediction of outcome in comatose survivors after cardiopulmonary resuscitation (an evidence-based review): report of the Quality Standards Subcommittee of the American Academy of Neurology. *Neurology* 2006; 67:203-210.

# Antidotes for the Intoxicated Patient

A 65-year-old man with history of undifferentiated liposarcoma was admitted to the oncology service for chemotherapy after being diagnosed with a recurrent abdominal mass. Chemotherapy consisted of adriamycin and ifosfamide. Two days later he developed confusion and multifocal jerks. We are called for a neurological evaluation and find the patient disoriented and delirious. When asked questions he perseverates, and his digit span is reduced to four. He can only recall 1 of 4 words after merely 3 minutes. Overall, he scores 19/30 points on the short-test for mental status examination. He has very frequent spontaneous multifocal myoclonus involving the face and all limbs. Some asterixis in the arms is also noted. There is no evidence of hyperreflexia, ataxia, or parkinsonism. None of the abnormal movements resemble seizures.

Because of concerns that the patient may be seizing or not be able to protect the airway, the patient is admitted to the intensive care unit.

*What do you do now?*

Our patient had clinical manifestations of ifosfamide toxicity and he responded well to the administration of 4 doses of methylene blue (50 mg intravenously every 6 hours). After 2 doses he was markedly better, and after 6 doses he had returned to baseline. It has been hypothesized that a metabolite of ifosfamide inhibits mitochondrial activity and this inhibition could be reversed by methylene blue, which facilitates electron transfer in the mitochondrial enzymatic respiratory chain. This case represents a dramatic example of the effects of an effective antidote for an acute intoxication affecting the central nervous system. However, these situations are not always so straightforward. Recognition of a specific intoxication and knowing what antidote to use can be major challenges for any physician. The differential diagnosis is usually extensive and baffling.

Neurologists are often involved because intoxications produce neurologic signs. Neurological presentations of intoxications are relatively nonspecific. Depressed level of consciousness (drowsiness, stupor, or even coma), altered content of consciousness (confusion, delusions, hallucinations), agitation, abnormal movements (myoclonus, asterixis, tremor), ataxia, rigidity, changes in deep tendon reflexes, and seizures can occur in various combinations depending on the type of toxin and the severity of the intoxication.

Clues to the toxic nature of the neurologic syndrome and even to the specific agent involved can be gathered from the history and the general physical examination. Knowledge of the physical manifestations of common toxidromes—syndromes caused by toxic agents—is therefore helpful to streamline management. Table 14.1 presents the most common toxidromes and the toxins that may cause them.

Perhaps the main reasons why we are consulted in the emergency department and medical ICU to evaluate intoxicated patients are coma and seizures. Table 14.2 lists the toxins that we have found most frequently associated with these neurological presentations. Several agents can produce coma and seizures in cases of severe intoxication. Therefore, in intoxicated comatose patients one should keep a low threshold for ordering electroencephalography to exclude nonconvulsive status epilepticus.

The treatment of these intoxicated patients depends greatly on the identification of the toxidrome and whether a specific antidote can be tried.

| Toxidrome | Manifestations | Agents |
|---|---|---|
| Anticholinergic syndrome | Delirium with hallucinations<br>Mydriasis<br>Hypertension<br>Tachycardia<br>Warm, dry, erythematous skin<br>Dry tongue and mucosas<br>Urinary retention<br>Seizures in most severe cases | Tricyclic antidepressants<br>Antihistamines<br>Antiparkinsonian medications<br>Antipsychotics<br>Belladonna alkaloids<br>Some mushrooms (e.g., *Amanita muscaria*) |
| Cholinergic syndrome | Confusion<br>Weakness and fasciculations<br>Miosis<br>Bradycardia<br>Diaphoresis<br>Salivation<br>Lacrimation<br>Diarrhea and cramping<br>Urinary incontinence<br>Seizures in most severe cases | Organophosphate insecticides<br>Pyridostigmine<br>Some mushrooms |
| Sympathetic syndrome | Delusions<br>Hyperreflexia<br>Mydriasis<br>Tachycardia<br>Hypertension<br>Fever<br>Diaphoresis and piloerection<br>Seizures in most severe cases | Cocaine<br>Amphetamines<br>Phencyclidine<br>Decongestants<br>Theophylline |
| Serotonin syndrome | Confusion or depressed consciousness<br>Tremor and akathisia<br>Myoclonus<br>Hyperreflexia/clonus (legs)<br>Rigidity (more in the legs)<br>Mydriasis<br>Tachycardia<br>Fever<br>Flushing<br>Diaphoresis<br>Diarrhea<br>Seizures in most severe cases | SSRI<br>Other antidepressants (e.g., venlafaxine, trazodone, buspirone)<br>MAO inhibitors<br>Opiates<br>Valproic acid<br>Triptans<br>Dextromethorphan<br>Metoclopramide<br>Linezolid<br>Lithium<br>St. John's wort<br>LSD, Ecstasy |

TABLE 14.1 **(Cont'd.)**

| Toxidrome | Manifestations | Agents |
|---|---|---|
| Ethanol intoxication | Hyperactive or hypoactive delirium progressing to coma<br>Tremors<br>Asterixis<br>Ataxia<br>Seizures<br>Tachycardia (possible arrhythmias)<br>Hypertension or hypotension<br>Vomiting | Ethanol |
| Atypical alcohol intoxication | Similar to ethanol, plus:<br>Severe acidosis with osmolal gap<br>Visual loss with methanol<br>Renal failure with ethylene glycol | Methanol<br>Ethylene glycol<br>Isopropyl alcohol |
| Opiate intoxication | Depressed consciousness<br>Hypoventilation<br>Miosis<br>Bradycardia<br>Hypotension<br>Hypothermia<br>Ileus<br>Seizures in most severe cases | All opiate agents |

SSRI, selective serotonin reuptake inhibitors; MAO, monoamino oxidase.


TABLE 14.2 **Causes to Consider in Coma and Seizures Due to Toxins**

| Coma | Seizures |
|---|---|
| Alcohols | Tricyclic antidepressants |
| Carbon monoxide | Cocaine |
| Benzodiazepines | Amphetamines |
| Opiates | Theophylline |
| Antidepressants (especially tricyclics) | Antiepileptics (overdose) |
| Antipsychotics | Opiates (especially meperidine) |
| Antihistamines | Baclofen |

*(Continues)*

TABLE 14.2 **(Cont'd.)**

| Coma | Seizures |
|---|---|
| Barbiturates | Beta-blockers |
| Other anticonvulsants | Clonidine |
| Other drugs of abuse | Hypoglycemic agents |
| Salicylates | Calcineurin inhibitors |
| Hypoglycemic agents | Other immunosuppressants (e.g., vincristine, cisplatin, intrathecal methotrexate) |

When no antidote is available, knowing which agent is involved will at least inform us about the chances of success of activated charcoal and the value of dialysis. Table 14.3 displays lists of toxic agents that bind well to activated charcoal, those that are cleared effectively with hemodialysis or hemoperfusion, and those that have a specific antidote. Unfortunately in cases of intentional overdoses, most patients have ingested several drugs instead of a single one. These cases are even more challenging not only in terms of diagnosis (a pure toxidrome is never clearly present) but also in terms of management because drug interactions may produce additional manifestations and complications.

Algorithms and lists are useful to keep around, but there are some caveats. Flumazenil lowers the seizures threshold and should not be used in patients with history of seizures or at high risk for having them. It is, therefore, unsafe to administer flumazenil in patients with suspected mixed overdoses which might include drugs that reduce seizure threshold. Naloxone and flumazenil are short-acting, so the improvement of the patients may be quite brief. Intubated patients should not be extubated while transiently more alert as many will lapse again into stupor and become once more unable to protect the airway. One should also be prepared to treat symptoms of acute opiate or benzodiazepine withdrawal when trying these medications. These agents are useful to prove the diagnosis and repeated doses can be used (continuous infusion of naloxone can be used as well), but they

| Good binding to activated charcoal* | Good clearance with dialysis | Good clearance with hemoperfusion | Antidotes** |
|---|---|---|---|
| Salicylates | Alcohols | Acetaminophen | Acetaminophen (Acetylcysteine) |
| Quinine | Barbiturates | Barbiturates | Benzodiazepines (Flumazenil) |
| Phenobarbital | Carbamazepine | Organophosphates | Opiates (Naloxone) |
| Carbamazepine | Valproic acid | Digoxin | Cyanide (Amyl nitrate) |
| Valproic acid | Amphetamines | Quinidine | Carbon monoxide (Oxygen, hyperbaric) |
| Phenytoin | MAO inhibitors | Theophylline | Methemoglobinemia (Methylene blue) |
| Diazepam | Beta-blockers | Methotrexate | Beta-blockers (Glucagon) |
| Digoxin | Lithium | | Digoxin (Digoxin-specific antibody fragments) |
| Theophilline | Salicylates | | |
| | Arsenic | | Arsenic (Dimercaprol) Mercury (N-acetylpenicillamine) |
| | Lead | | Copper (Penicillamine) |
| | | | Organophosphates (Neostigmine, oximes) |
| | | | Ifosfamide (Methylene blue) |

MAO, monoamino oxidase.
*Evidence from comparative studies is often lacking.
**Antidote in parentheses.

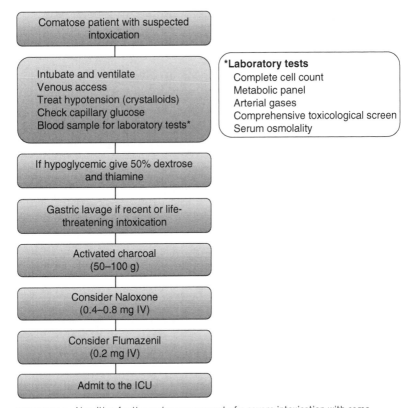

FIGURE 14.1 Algorithm for the early management of a severe intoxication with coma.

do not eliminate the toxin and therefore do not solve the problem. Supportive therapy is needed for severe opiate and benzodiazepine intoxications to resolve.

The management of a severe intoxication may be complex and requires a comprehensive game plan. Figure 14.1 presents an algorithm of the initial management of severe intoxications. Poor outcome may be due to the initial effects of the toxin or due to secondary complications, such as poor oxygenation and shock. However aggressive supportive care is warranted in almost all patients. The irony, of course, is that most self-intoxicated patients actually want to recover.

- Intoxications often present with prominent neurological features, most notably depressed consciousness, delirium, abnormal movements, and seizures. None of these manifestations are specific for any single toxin.
- Recognition of the most common toxidromes can guide management and predict complications.
- Early management focuses on securing the airway, ensuring adequate oxygenation, achieving hemodynamic stabilization, excluding hypoglycemia, and considering gastrointestinal decontamination. Antidotes (such as naloxone, flumazenil) may be administered in appropriate cases.
- Naloxone and flumazenil may be very effective, but their effects are short-lasting.

### Further Reading

Betten DP, Vohra RB, Cook MD, Matteucci MJ, Clark RF. Antidote use in the critically ill poisoned patient. *J Intensive Care Med* 2006; 21:255-277.

Bond GR. The role of activated charcoal and gastric emptying in gastrointestinal decontamination: a state-of-the-art review. *Ann Emerg Med* 2002; 39:273-286.

Boyer EW, Shannon M. The serotonin syndrome. *N Engl J Med* 2005; 352:1112-1120.

Hoffman RS, Goldfrank LR. The poisoned patient with altered consciousness: controversies in the use of a "coma cocktail." *JAMA* 1995; 274:562-569.

Meehan TJ, Bryant SM, Aks SE. Drugs of abuse: the highs and lows of altered mental states in the emergency department. *Emerg Med Clin North Am*. 2010:28: 663-683.

Patel PN. Methylene blue for management of ifosfamide-induced encephalopathy. *Ann Pharmacother* 2006; 40:299-303.

Wijdicks EFM. *The Comatose Patient*. Oxford University Press, New York, 2008.

# Failure to Awaken After Surgery

A 56-year-old woman with prior polysubstance abuse underwent emergent repair of a perforated duodenal ulcer. Surgery was uncomplicated with no major blood loss or marked hypotension. Following surgery, the patient was initially agitated and thought to be in a withdrawal delirium. She received several doses of lorazepam. This resulted in calm behavior, but she continued to "wake up slowly." The surgical intensive care service noted that she did not speak and barely responded to voice. Several days later, she was found to have "unintelligible" speech.

Neurology was consulted, and on our examination the patient has a markedly dysarthric speech, limited upgaze, and vertical nystagmus. There is a severe appendicular dysmetria. A CT scan was immediately ordered and it shows acute bilateral cerebellar hypodensities and acute hydrocephalus (Figure 15.1).

*What do you do now?*

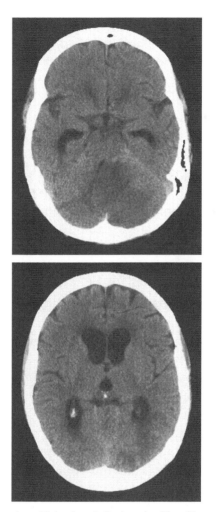

**FIGURE 15.1** CT scan shows bilateral cerebellar hypodensities with acute obstructive hydrocephalus.

Without doubt, abnormal wakefulness after a surgical procedure is the most common reason for neurological consultation in surgical intensive care units. The ambiguous- and unfortunately pervasive-term "altered mental status" is typically used to characterize patients who are not fully awake following a major surgical repair, and who do not respond well to the surgeon's questions during rounds.

There are a few obvious causes. Complex cardiac or vascular procedures are most often associated with ischemic brain lesions. Most surgeons anticipate "trouble ahead" when mobile atherosclerotic plaques are found or prolonged hypotension has occurred during major vascular surgery, and both are strong indicators the brain could have been affected.

Ischemic stroke involving major arterial territories are expected in any type of vascular surgery, such as aortic arch replacement, surgery for aortic dissection, or any type of open-heart surgery. Strokes in the cerebellum can be explained by a vertebral occlusion (e.g., dissecting aorta occluding the vertebral artery origins), but the posterior circulation is often involved in cardiogenic stroke (postoperative myocardial infarction and new postoperative atrial fibrillation are known contenders). The diagnostic yield of MRI scan in a patient who remains stuporous can be substantial, and MRI can show multiple hemispheric lesions that may explain failure to awaken after anesthesia.

Multiple cases of postoperative stupor associated with bithalamic infarcts have been described. Therefore, MRI/MRA is essential in postoperative patients in whom sedation cannot explain the decreased level of consciousness.

In patients undergoing a general (nonvascular-noncardiac) surgical procedure—as in our case example—neurologic complications are not expected. Multiple ischemic strokes after a general surgical procedure (defined as urogenital, gastrointestinal, orthopedic, or chest surgery) without involving some sort of manipulation of vasculature is rare and hard to explain. It occurs most often in patients who have other stroke risk factors, such as peripheral vascular disease or ischemic cardiomyopathy. Hypotension does not play a major role unless an unexpected large blood loss has occurred. When ischemic stroke involves the posterior circulation resulting in cerebellar infarcts with obstructive hydrocephalus (explaining stupor), the diagnosis is difficult and often not recognized. This was clearly the case in our patient. Following any type of surgery, there is a tendency for strokes to occur in the posterior circulation territories, and therefore, it has been speculated that these strokes could be due to vertebral dissection occurring as a result of neck manipulation associated with anesthesia preparation. No such case has ever been documented to corroborate that explanation. In our patient example, the sudden appearance of a bilateral cerebellar infarct compressing the fourth ventricle led to an obstructive hydrocephalus.

After ventriculostomy was placed, the patient improved substantially, and eventually the ventriculostomy was weaned and removed.

Finally, it is worth emphasizing that the cause of postoperative stupor in general surgical intensive care units usually is due to prolonged clearance of sedative drugs or excessive opioid use. The additional presence of multiorgan failure in critically ill patients may reduce clearance of any of these drugs, and a careful look at the medication dose, infusion rate, and expected clearance is necessary. Increased creatinine after cardiac surgery is a major determinant of prolonged awakening after cardiac surgery.

Also rare, but often considered a diagnostic possibility, is the presence of nonconvulsive status epilepticus. This is a highly unusual occurrence after any type of surgical procedure or in any critical illness. It can occur more often in patients who have had seizures or in patients who had a known seizure disorder and did not have their antiepileptic drugs administered.

Acute metabolic derangement such as acute hyponatremia or acute hyperglycemia are always considered and, occasionally, these derangements explain the clinical picture. In susceptible patients a surgical procedure may lead to an acute increase in serum ammonia (mostly young females in teenage years with an ornithine transcarbamylase deficiency or in patients after a lung transplantation).

TABLE 15.1 **Causes to Consider in Patients Who Fail to Awaken after Surgery**

Excessive opioid use

Prolonged clearance of benzodiazepines with multiorgan failure

Postoperative stroke (hemisphere with mass effect)

Postoperative stroke (cerebellum with mass effect or hydrocephalus)

Postoperative PRES (aortic dissection repair)

Acute hyponatremia

Acute hypoglycemia or hyperglycemia

Acute hypercapnia with hypoxemia

Acute uremia

Acute increase in arterial ammonia

Nonconvulsive status epilepticus

PRES: Posterior reversible encephalopathy syndrome.

So the next time you are asked to see a patient with postoperative stupor in the surgical ICU with "altered mental status" think sedatives, stroke, seizures, or a sudden metabolic derangement. But frankly, the 3 major causes of failure to awaken postoperatively are drugs, drugs and drugs (even if everyone denies it).

## KEY POINTS TO REMEMBER REGARDING FAILURE TO AWAKEN AFTER SURGERY

- Postoperative stupor is usually associated with excessive sedation. As a general rule, the expected clearance of an opioid or benzodiazepine is usually five times its half-life.
- In stuporous patients, consider an ischemic stroke in the posterior circulation involving the thalamus or cerebellar infarctions causing acute hydrocephalus from compression.
- Hyponatremia and hypoglycemia are potential causes of postoperative stupor. Hypoglycemia requires immediate correction, while hyponatremia should be corrected more slowly.

### Further Reading

Limburg M, Wijdicks EFM, Li H. Ischemic stroke after surgical procedures: clinical features, neuroimaging, and risk factors. *Neurology* 1998; 50:895-901.

Sinclair RCF. Delayed recovery of consciousness after anesthesia. *Br J Anesth: CEACCP* 2006; 3: 114-118.

Rodriquez RA, Bussière M, Bourke M. Predictors of duration of unconsciousness in patients with coma after cardiac surgery. J *Cardiothoracic Vasc Anesth* 2011, ahead of print.

Stevens RD, Nyquist PA. Coma, delirium, and cognitive dysfunction in critical illness. *Crit Care Clin*. 2008; 22:787-804.

Wijdicks EFM. Neurologic complications in critically ill patients. *Anesth Analg* 1996; 83: 411-419.

# Stupor After Brain Surgery

A 23-year-old man presents with a syncopal event and during evaluation was found to have a tumor in the posterior fossa. He underwent surgical resection of a tumor filling the fourth ventricle extending into the cerebellopontine angle and upper cervical spinal canal (Figure 16.1A). Pathology showed WHO grade II ependymoma. Following surgery the patient had dysarthria, dysphagia, and left hemi-ataxia. On the second day of surgery he underwent a reexploration with removal of an extradural hematoma in the posterior fossa and recovered well. A week later, he unexpectedly became gradually more stuporous, developed a new hemiparesis, and was transferred back to the neurosciences intensive care unit. On examination, he was not following simple commands, looked about, was mute and grinded his teeth. He had an increased snout reflex and bilateral grasp reflexes. His brainstem reflexes were intact. He had considerable right arm weakness barely overcoming gravity. CT scan showed new appearance of multiple hemispheric hypodensities, largely in the posterior frontal lobes (Figure 16.1B). His laboratory studies were normal. Cerebral angiogram shows diffuse cerebral vasospasm in both anterior and posterior circulation (Figure 16.1C).

*What do you do now?*

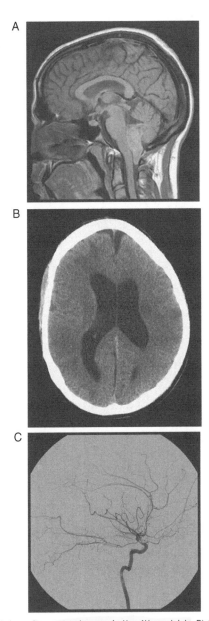

**FIGURE 16.1** A) MRI shows large ependymona in the 4th ventricle. B) CT scan about 10 days after surgery shows multiple hypodensities. C) The cerebral angiogram (sample of multiple series) shows cerebral vasospasm in the anterior circulation.

In order to detect deterioration patients undergoing elective brain tumor surgery are commonly observed overnight in an intensive or intermediate care unit. Most patients will leave the intensive care unit without any complications. When neurointensivists are asked by neurosurgeons to become involved in postoperative care it is because the current clinical condition is unexplained and unusual, because seizures have occurred, or because a major systemic complication needs very close attention. Complications after craniotomy are relatively uncommon but may be more frequent after extensive and complex neurosurgery. To give some sense of what to consider, Table 16.1 lists several causes of deterioration after a craniotomy.

Any patient with an early deterioration may be having seizures, but most patients who are stuporous or comatose from seizures will have already shown focal twitches that then became more generalized and evolved into a nonconvulsive status epilepticus. The cause may not be clear or simply related to removal of brain tumor tissue. Best treatment options in these patients include intravenous levetiracetam loading with 1500–2000 mg or intravenous loading with 20 mg per kg of (fos) phenytoin.

Postoperative hemorrhage in the operative bed may or may not be symptomatic. When mass effect occurs, patients are more likely to decline. A more recently identified cause of neurologic deterioration is the appearance of a hematoma remote from the surgical site. These surprising venous hemorrhages may be in the opposite hemisphere or in the cerebellum in patients with surgery of cerebral hemispheres. It may also occur after drainage of an acute subdural hematoma. The mechanism is therefore most likely mechanical shift of the brain ("sagging") after reducing intracranial pressure. These remote hemorrhages can become clinically relevant and because they are lobar in nature may actually present with new seizures. Hemorrhage in

TABLE 16.1 **Causes of Deterioration after Craniotomy**

Seizures (partial or generalized) and status epilepticus
Postoperative hemorrhage (operative bed or remote)
Cerebral infarction (sacrifice of an arterial branch or cerebral vein)
Postoperative cerebral edema
Diffuse cerebral vasospasm
Medical complications (e.g., hyponatremia or hypernatremia after
   pituitary surgery)

the cerebellar peduncles have produced new onset slurred speech, tremor, cerebellar ataxia, and nystagmus. Most of the time, these hemorrhages resolve on their own, and the impact on outcome is not substantial.

Cerebral infarction can occur after craniotomy when there is sacrifice of an arterial or venous branch, and the typical example is a sizable meningioma extirpation with necessary sacrifice of large venous tributaries.

Some neurosurgical procedures have the potential for more specific complications in the postoperative days. These include patients with epilepsy surgery who have hemorrhagic complications associated with depth electrode placement and patients after pituitary surgery with major adrenal or thyroid deficiencies. Hyponatremia may occur after several days and may be profound. Hypernatremia may follow hyponatremia, and even a triphasic postoperative course (hypernatremia–hyponatremia–hypernatremia) may occur. Large amounts of fluids and marked decline in vasopressin levels may contribute. (see chapter 26)

Our patient had a postoperative complication that is well described, probably more common than appreciated, but rarely considered. Obviously, cerebral vasospasm is not recognized unless a cerebral angiogram is performed. Early on, even an MR angiogram may not be sufficiently sensitive to demonstrate vasospasm that starts in smaller arterial branches. The onset of new neurologic signs, particularly when not easily grouped into a single syndrome and the appearance of new onset multifocal ischemia on CT scan should point toward this possibility. In prior reported patients the diffuse cerebral vasospasm occured several days and up to a week after surgery, and its development was associated with clear clinical deterioration. Patients may have fluctuating neurologic deficits that could point toward the diagnosis. Cerebral vasospasm may be more prevalent in certain types of neurosurgical procedures and in particular after skull base surgery. A commonly implicated surgery is pituitary adenoma resection via transcranial or transsphenoidal approach.

The pathophysiology of cerebral vasospasm after tumor surgery is not known. Removal of tumor adjacent to the basal cisterns could release vasoactive substances, but this remains speculative. Intraoperative hemorrhage and postoperative blood on the subarachnoid cisterns were not prominent in reported cases and have not been factors in the cases we have seen. Mechanical manipulation with extensive mobilization of medium size arteries during surgery might be another cause. Yet, this does not explain the diffuse distribution of the vasospasm or its development after a prolonged interval. Therefore, neither what we know about delayed vasospasm following aneurysmal subarachnoid hemorrhage nor what we know about reversible cerebral vasoconstriction syndrome appears to apply well to these cases of vasospasm after brain tumor surgery.

After the diagnosis is established there is uncertainty on how to best approach and treat this condition. If the situation allows, the treatment should be 1) increase cerebral perfusion by opening up the larger arteries through angioplasty and 2) increase cerebral perfusion pressure with traditional methods of hemodynamic augmentation.

In our patient, there was significant diffuse cerebral vasospasm that warranted immediate balloon angioplasty and intra-arterial infusion of verapamil in multiple arterial segments. He was additionally treated with aggressive hemodynamic augmentation using vasopressors and albumin, and with calcium channel blockers. He recovered gradually and eventually achieved an acceptable functional outcome.

Even if unusual, it is important to consider cerebral vasospasm after brain surgery in any patient with unexplained deterioration because endovascular intervention is indicated and successful if done early.

---

**KEY POINTS TO REMEMBER REGARDING STUPOR AFTER BRAIN SURGERY**

- Neurological worsening after craniotomy for tumor surgery can be due to cerebral vasospasm. The cerebral vasospasm can be diffuse and not only in the surgical field and may only be documented by cerebral angiogram.
- Worsening can also occur because of hemorrhage in the surgical bed, remote hemorrhage, cerebral edema, or ischemic stroke from sacrifice of a large vein or artery.
- Postoperative seizures may present with focal seizures, which may evolve into partial or generalized status epilepticus.

**Further Reading**

Almubaslat M, Africk C. Cerebral vasospasm after resection of an esthesioneuroblastoma: case report and literature review. *Surg Neurol* 2007; 68:322-328.

Amini A, Osborn AG, McCall TD, Couldwell WT. Remote cerebellar hemorrhage. *AJNR Am J Neuroradiol* 2006; 27:387-390.

Bejjani GD, Sekhar LN, Yost AM, Bank WO, Wright DC. Vasospasm after cranial base tumor resection: pathogenesis, diagnosis, and therapy. *Surg Neurol* 1999; 52:577-583.

Brockmann MA, Groden C. Remote cerebellar hemorrhage: a review. *Cerebellum.* 2006;5:64-68.

LeRoux PD, Haglund MM, Mayberg MR, Winn HR. Symptomatic cerebral vasospasm following tumor resection: report of two cases. *Surg Neurol* 1991; 36:25-31.

# Calls, Pages, and Other Alarms

# Acute Delirium

A 72-year-old man with history of hypertension, diabetes mellitus, and a right subcortical ischemic stroke three years before was admitted with acute abdominal pain. Exploratory laparotomy revealed perforated diverticulitis. He underwent partial colectomy and colostomy without complications. In the surgical ICU he was treated with fluids, vasopressors, and antibiotics for sepsis. Complications included acute kidney injury and mild elevation of liver transaminases. He was kept on mechanical ventilation and sedated with a midazolam infusion. Three days after the surgery we are consulted because the patient is agitated every time the nurses try to diminish the sedation. On examination he fluctuates between drowsiness and agitation and he has multifocal adventitious movements.

**What do you do now?**

D elirium is a very common complication in the ICU. It can follow critical medical or surgical illness. It may be seen in 15% to 80% of critically ill patients depending on the severity of the underlying illness, the age, and the previous cognitive status. Another factor that explains the wide variation of reported rates of ICU delirium is that it is often underrecognized. Some clinicians seem to accept a certain degree of drowsiness, agitation, or confusion in elderly critically ill patients. However, delirium is a form of brain dysfunction associated with poor clinical outcomes and potentially persistent cognitive decline.

The raving, raging patient is obvious, but many patients with ICU delirium do not have pure or even predominant hyperactivity. Instead, mixed and hypoactive forms of delirium are more common. Monitoring tools sensitive to hyperactive and hypoactive manifestations of delirium have to be used to prevent cases from going unnoticed. Using a validated scale for monitoring the level of sedation, such as the Richmond Agitation Sedation Scale (RASS) (Table 17.1), is advisable.

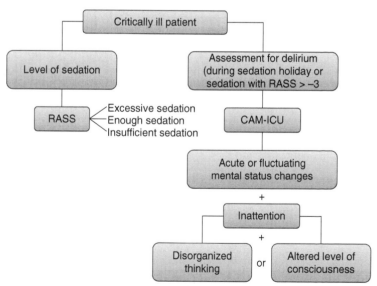

FIGURE 17.1 Assessment of level of sedation and delirium in the ICU. RASS, Richmond Agitation Sedation Scale (see Table 17.3); CAM-ICU, Confusion Assessment Method for the ICU: delirium is diagnosed by the presence of 3 of the 4 diagnostic features.

TABLE 17.1 **The Richmond Agitation Sedation Scale for the Assessment of Depth of Sedation**

| | |
|---|---|
| +4 | Very combative, violent, dangerous to staff |
| +3 | Pulling catheters and tubes, aggressive |
| +2 | Frequent nonpurposeful movements, fights ventilator |
| +1 | Anxious but movements not aggressive or vigorous |
| 0 | Alert and calm |
| -1 | Awakes (eye contact) for > 10 seconds in response to voice |
| -2 | Awakes (eye contact) for < 10 seconds in response to voice |
| -3 | Eye opening or movement to voice without eye contact |
| -4 | No response to voice, but eye opening or movement to physical stimulation |
| -5 | No response to voice or physical stimulation |

Sedation holidays (stopping all sedatives at regular intervals) have been shown to decrease the duration of mechanical ventilation and the length of ICU stay. They also decrease the incidence of delirium. Still, the need for sedation holidays is not sufficiently appreciated. In fact, it has been our experience that precisely the sickest patient is the one at highest risk for delirium and in whom sedation holidays are less frequently used.

We still know little about the causes and mechanisms of delirium in critically ill patients, but there is emerging research. Studies have definitively demonstrated that prolonged exposure to psychoactive drugs in general and sedative drugs in particular increase the risk and severity of delirium. Benzodiazepines are particularly prone to exacerbate delirium and they are only indicated for the treatment of delirium related to alcohol withdrawal. Dexmedetomidine may be a safer option. Antidopaminergic agents are the best medications for agitation; the relative value of haloperidol versus atypical antipsychotics (such quetiapine or olanzepine) is not well studied in the ICU population. The risk of delirium with opiates has been less studied, but we often find them to be a major contributing factor. The general principle is that we should be using all sedatives very judiciously, prescribing the lowest possible doses and stopping them as soon as they are no longer truly necessary. In fact, a good first step would be to ensure that we avoid sedating critically ill patients who are already drowsy (when not stuporous or comatose), an everyday error in many ICUs today.

As neurologists we are often consulted to evaluate these patients in the medical or the surgical ICU and we can be very useful. Table 17.2 lists some of the diagnoses to consider when evaluating "encephalopathic" patients in general ICUs. The experienced clinician will look for brainstem or lateralizing signs, subtle manifestations of seizures, and features of major toxidromes (see chapter 14). Adventitious movements such as multifocal myoclonus (more common with uremia) and asterixis (more common with liver failure) are good markers of a metabolic derangement, albeit nonspecific. Severe muscle rigidity with clonus should raise suspicion for serotonin syndrome, neuroleptic malignant syndrome, and when accompanied by high fever, malignant hyperthermia.

Our approach to the evaluation of patients with ICU delirium is summarized in Table 17.3. In essence, after reviewing the history and examining the patient, we try to answer the following questions:

- Do I have a diagnosis?
- Should the patient have more blood tests?
- Should the patient have brain imaging? If so, which one?
- Should the patient have a lumbar puncture?
- Should the patient have an electroencephalogram? If so, is there a need for continuous monitoring?
- Are there any medications in the regimen that should be reduced or stopped?
- Do I need to recommend specific treatment for agitation?

In the case presented, we found that the patient had mixed delirium with multifocal myoclonus, but normal brainstem reflexes and no lateralizing signs on examination. Muscle tone was normal. Deep tendon reflexes were decreased in the legs, consistent with his long history of diabetes. He had no meningeal signs or clinical manifestations of seizures. We requested a serum ammonia level, which was normal, and decided to follow his clinical evolution without recommending further testing. We did ask the primary team to stop the infusion of midazolam and to use intravenous haloperidol (2–5 mg every 4 hours) for the patient's episodic agitation.

TABLE 17.2  **Differential Diagnoses in ICU Patients with Encephalopathy**

| Diagnosis | Signs | Test | Intervention |
|---|---|---|---|
| Meningitis | Neck rigidity<br>Kernig sign<br>Brudzinski sign | Lumbar puncture | Antimicrobials |
| Encephalitis | +/- lateralizing signs<br>+/- seizures | Lumbar puncture | Acyclovir if HSV<br>Gancyclovir if CMV<br>Antiepileptic drugs if seizures<br>Supportive care otherwise |
| Status epilepticus | Abnormal eye movements<br>Rhythmic movements in the extremities<br>Facial automatisms<br>Staring | EEG | Antiepileptic drugs |
| Ischemic stroke | Lateralizing signs (right parietal, multifocal)<br>Brainstem signs (basilar artery occlusion) | Neuroimaging | Reperfusion if acute<br>Evaluate mechanism<br>Secondary prevention |
| Intracranial hemorrhage | Lateralizing signs | Neuroimaging | Consider neuro-surgery consult |
| Dural venous sinus thrombosis | Lateralizing signs | CTV, MRV | Anticoagulation<br>Consider endovascular therapy when worsening |
| Fat embolism syndrome | Acute agitation<br>Conjunctival ecchymoses<br>+/- lateralizing signs | Neuroimaging | Supportive<br>Avoid manipulating the fracture<br>Evaluate for patent foramen ovale |
| Neuroleptic malignant syndrome | Extreme rigidity<br>Fever<br>Autonomic instability | Serum CK | Stop antidopaminergics<br>Consider dantrolene |
| Serotonin syndrome | Rigidity, tremor<br>Hyperreflexia, clonus<br>Mydriasis<br>Autonomic instability | Serum CK | Stop serotonergic drugs<br>Consider cyproheptadine |

(*Continues*)

TABLE 17.2  **(Cont'd.)**

| Diagnosis | Signs | Test | Intervention |
|---|---|---|---|
| Malignant hyperthermia* | Very high fever Autonomic instability Severe rigidity Hyporeflexia | Arterial blood gas Lactic acid Serum CK | Aggressive control of fever Treatment of acidosis Dantrolene |
| Anticholinergic toxicity | Mydriasis Skin dry, erythematous. Dry tongue and mucosa. Tachycardia Ileus | | Removal of culprit drug |
| Alcohol withdrawal† | Tremor Diaphoresis Tachycardia +/- seizures | - | Benzodiazepines Thiamine Electrolyte replacement |
| Uremic encephal- opathy | Prominent multifocal myoclonus Tremor Hyperreflexia (if no severe peripheral neuropathy) | Serum BUN | Dialysis if necessary |
| Hepatic encephal- opathy | Prominent asterixis Tremor Often ataxia | Serum ammonia | Lactulose Rifaximin |
| ICU delirium | Nothing specific | | Minimize sedatives and opiates Haloperidol or atypical antipsychotics for agitation General supportive care |

*Only within 30 minutes to 24 hours after exposure to inhalational anesthesia or succinylcholine.
† Presented as an example of drug withdrawal syndrome.
BUN, blood urea nitrogen; CK, creatine kinase; CTV, CT venography; CMV, cytomegalovirus; EEG, electroencephalogram; HSV, herpes virus simplex; MRV, magnetic resonance venography

**TABLE 17.3  Approach to the Patient with ICU Delirium**

| Evaluation | Indication |
|---|---|
| History (including preadmission functional and cognitive status) | All patients |
| Physical examination | All patients |
| Blood tests | Metabolic panel including BUN, liver transaminases, and serum ammonia in all cases. CK level if rigidity. Lactic acid if sepsis or acidosis. Toxicological screen in any case of coma or delirium at presentation with no known cause. |
| Brain imaging | If lateralizing signs, brainstem signs. |
| Lumbar puncture | Unexplained fever/sepsis. Meningeal signs. |
| Electroencephalogram | Rhythmic abnormal movements. Staring, not tracking finger. Consider in any case of unexplained coma. |

We also strongly advised to stop the infusion of fentanyl that the patient had been receiving since surgery. With these simple changes, the patient began to improve despite further increase in his BUN for two more days (to reach a peak of 58 mg/dL) before it started to decline. Once off sedatives, he was extubated without complications. Upon discharge 2 weeks later, his intellectual function was nearly normal.

The evaluation of delirium may seem overwhelming, but a simple checklist including the questions listed above may help avoid oversights and focus the consultation.

---

**KEY POINTS TO REMEMBER REGARDING ACUTE DELIRIUM**

- Altered level and content of consciousness is never a normal finding in a patient in the ICU. If present, it deserves careful attention.
- ICU delirium is a common complication of medical and surgical critical illness and it is associated with worse short-term and long-term clinical outcomes.

- Delirium does not always mean agitation. Some patients with delirium are actually hypoactive.
- Standardized tools, such as the CAM-ICU score, should be used for the timely recognition of ICU delirium.
- Sedatives (especially benzodiazepines) and opiates worsen delirium, and their use should be minimized as much as possible.
- Always exclude primary neurological diseases in any critical patient with evidence of brain dysfunction.

### Further Reading

Ely EW, Inouye SK, Bernard GR, Gordon S, Francis J, May L, Truman B, Speroff T, Gautam S, Margolin R, Hart RP, Dittus R. Delirium in mechanically ventilated patients: validity and reliability of the confusion assessment method for the intensive care unit (CAM-ICU). *JAMA* 2001; 286:2703-2710.

Ely EW, Truman B, Shintani A, Thomason JW, Wheeler AP, Gordon S, Francis J, Speroff T, Gautam S, Margolin R, Sessler CN, Dittus RS, Bernard GR. Monitoring sedation status over time in ICU patients: reliability and validity of the Richmond Agitation-Sedation Scale (RASS). *JAMA* 2003; 289:2983-2991.

Frontera JA. Delirium and sedation in the ICU. *Neurocrit Care.* 2011;14:463-474.

Girard TD, Jackson JC, Pandharipande PP, Pun BT, Thompson JL, Shintani AK, Gordon SM, Canonico AE, Dittus RS, Bernard GR, Ely EW. Delirium as a predictor of long-term cognitive impairment in survivors of critical illness. *Crit Care Med* 2010; 38:1513-1520.

Girard TD, Pandharipande PP, Ely EW. Delirium in the intensive care unit. *Crit Care* 2008; 12 Suppl 3:S3.

Jacobi J, Fraser GL, Coursin DB, Riker RR, Fontaine D, Wittbrodt ET, Chalfin DB, Masica MF, Bjerke HS, Coplin WM, Crippen DW, Fuchs BD, Kelleher RM, Marik PE, Nasraway SA Jr, Murray MJ, Peruzzi WT, Lumb PD; Task Force of the American College of Critical Care Medicine (ACCM) of the Society of Critical Care Medicine (SCCM), American Society of Health-System Pharmacists (ASHP), American College of Chest Physicians. Clinical practice guidelines for the sustained use of sedatives and analgesics in the critically ill adult. *Crit Care Med* 2002; 30:119-141.

Kress JP, Pohlman AS, O'Connor MF, Hall JB . Daily interruption of sedative infusions in critically ill patients undergoing mechanical ventilation. *N Engl J Med* 2000; 342:1471-1477.

Pandharipande PP, Pun BT, Herr DL, Maze M, Girard TD, Miller RR, Shintani AK, Thompson JL, Jackson JC, Deppen SA, Stiles RA, Dittus RS, Bernard GR, Ely EW. Effect of sedation with dexmedetomidine vs lorazepam on acute brain dysfunction in mechanically ventilated patients: the MENDS randomized controlled trial. *JAMA* 2007; 298:2644-2653.

Wong CL, Holroyd-Leduc J, Simel DL, Straus SE. Does this patient have delirium? value of bedside instruments. *JAMA.* 2010;304:779-786.

A 50-year-old man with history of hypertension, heavy
smoking, and alcoholism was admitted with poor-grade
subarachnoid hemorrhage (WFNS grade IV). Cerebral
angiogram showed an anterior communicating artery
aneurysm, which was successfully coiled. His condition
improved after placement of a ventriculostomy catheter,
but shortly thereafter his level and content of
consciousness started to fluctuate because of alcohol
withdrawal. Despite treatment with benzodiazepines
and dexmedetomidine, he had frequent episodes of
agitation, diaphoresis, hyperthermia, and tachycardia.
He remained intubated and mechanically ventilated.
Serial transcranial Doppler measurements showed
progressively increasing mean blood flow velocities
in the anterior and middle cerebral arteries bilaterally
starting on post bleeding day 6. On day 8, a CT
angiogram confirmed the presence of mild to moderate
diffuse vasospasm, but with normal mean transit time
and cerebral blood flow on the CT perfusion. On post

bleeding days 10 and 11 he was responding better to commands. However, a day later he suddenly developed a fever of 40 degrees Celsius and became abruptly hypotensive. He is again stuporous.

M ajor medical complications can be expected in any mechanically ventilated patient with an acute brain injury, and they may come suddenly. Basically, acute fever and hypotension—manifestations of systemic inflammatory response syndrome (Table 18.1)—should always trigger immediate activation of the sepsis management protocol. Any delays can be problematic, even more so in patients with possible compromise of cerebral perfusion. The general principles of management of septic shock apply to patients with acute brain injury (Table 18.2).

In critically ill neurologic patients certain aspects of care may have to be adjusted. Aggressive fluid resuscitation should be started emergently with 1000–2000 mL of crystalloids over 30 minutes. In patients with cerebral edema we think that normal saline is preferable to lactated Ringer to avoid fluids with lower tonicity. Colloids (albumin) can also be used. The usual set target in the treatment of sepsis is a mean arterial pressure of 65 mmHg, but a higher target may be necessary in patients at risk of cerebral ischemia. Serum lactate should be measured quickly and it is an important indicator of the seriousness of the situation. A serum lactic acid level > 4 mmol/L indicates tissue hypoperfusion and calls for aggressive hemodynamic support. The patient's urinary output needs to be closely monitored for the development of oliguria (less than 20 ml/hour). Goal-directed therapy within the first 6 hours (aiming for a central venous oxygen saturation ≥ 70%) may reduce mortality. Norepinephrine is the initial vasopressor of choice. It may be supplemented with low dose vasopressin (0.04 units per minute) if the blood pressure target is not achieved. Epinephrine and dopamine are reasonable options. However, the pure alpha adrenergic agonist phenylephrine is not a good choice in septic shock because it can reduce cardiac output

TABLE 18.1 **Systemic Inflammatory Response Syndrome (SIRS)***

| Physiological variable | Measurement |
| --- | --- |
| Body temperature | > 38.5-°C or < 35°C |
| Heart rate | > 90 beats per minute |
| Respiratory rate | > 20 breaths per minute or $PaCO_2$ < 32 mmHg |
| White blood cell count | > 12,000 cells/mm³, 4,000 cells/mm³, or > 10% bands |

* SIRS with proven infection defines sepsis.

TABLE 18.2 **Initial Treatment of Septic Shock with Special Considerations in Neurological Patients**

*Start aggressive fluid resuscitation immediately*
1-2 liters of 0.9% NaCl (may add intermittent infusions of 250 cc of albumin 5%)

*Define resuscitation goal*
A MAP goal higher than the usual 65 mmHg may be necessary in neurocritical
    patients with compromised cerebral perfusion

*Start vasopressor if MAP below target after fluid challenge*
Norepinephrine, low dose vasopressin, epinephrine
Phenylephrine is not adequate

*Obtain echocardiogram and assess systolic function*
Start dobutamine if decreased left ventricular ejection fraction

*Conservative fluid strategy after resuscitation goal is achieved*
Can use diuretics if MAP stable and evidence of cerebral edema or raised ICP

*Diagnosis of infectious source*
Panculture (blood cultures, urinalysis with culture and sensitivity,
    sputum sample)
Culture CSF

*Start broad-spectrum antibiotics as soon as possible*

*Consider hydrocortisone if vasopressor dependence*

*Avoid activated human recombinant protein C if increased risk of ICH*

*Blood product administration*
Consider red blood cell transfusion to keep hemoglobin > 9-10 g/dL if
    cerebral perfusion is compromised
Platelet transfusion to keep platelet count > 50,000 if recent ICH or neurosurgery
FFP to correct coagulopathy if recent ICH or neurosurgery

*Mechanical ventilation*
Careful titration of PEEP if raised ICP

*Sedation and analgesia*
Sedation holidays
Minimize use of opiates if possible

*Glucose control*
Maintain blood sugars between 140-180 mg/dL

MAP, mean arterial pressure; CSF, cerebrospinal fluid; ICH, intracranial hemorrhage; FFP, fresh
    frozen plasma; PEEP, positive end expiratory pressure; ICP, intracranial pressure

(i.e., stroke volume) and patients with sepsis may already have myocardial dysfunction. In fact, these patients should have an urgent echocardiogram. If the left ventricular ejection fraction is reduced and shock persists, dobutamine—an inotropic agent—should be started. After the patient has been successfully resuscitated, fluid administration must be very conservative (i.e., fluid balance even to negative) to prevent complications from fluid overload (principally related to capillary leak leading to pulmonary edema). However, this approach can create a dilemma in certain acute neurological disorders. In patients with brain edema, maintaining a negative fluid balance is actually desirable. Instead, patients with symptomatic vasospasm can become ischemic if they develop intravascular volume contraction.

Patients with refractory septic shock may be treated with corticosteroids (hydrocortisone 50 mg intravenously every 6 hours). Corticosteroids may reduce vasopressor dependency but do not appear to improve survival. Their use should not be a problem in critical neurological patients. However, recombinant human activated protein C must not be administered to patients with intracranial hemorrhage or recent neurosurgery, because there is an increased risk of hemorrhage associated with the use of this drug.

Early initiation of broad-spectrum antibiotics is crucially important. Ideally, they should be started within the first hour of the diagnosis of septic shock. Pancultures should be obtained before the first antibiotic dose if at all possible, but cannot delay the start of antibiotics. Nosocomial meningitis may be associated with early sepsis, and thus cultures should include a cerebrospinal fluid sample in any patient with cerebrospinal fluid diversion devices (ventriculostomy, lumbar drainage) or previous neurosurgical procedures.

Septic shock guidelines generally recommend transfusion of red blood cells only when the hemoglobin concentration is below 7 g/dL. While we still do not know the ideal hemoglobin target in patients with severe acute brain insults, such as severe traumatic head injury or poor-grade subarachnoid hemorrhage, improving oxygen carrying capacity may be particularly beneficial in these patients with compromised cerebral perfusion and recent or persistent hypotension. Until more information is available, we aim at a higher target of hemoglobin concentration of 9–10 g/dL in critically ill neurological patients who are septic and hypotensive.

Glucose management should also be more cautious in patients with acute brain injury. Cerebral microdialysis studies have shown that neuroglycopenia and anaerobic metabolism can occur with glycemias between 60–80 mg/dL, which are levels often considered acceptable in other patients. We use insulin infusions in hyperglycemic patients but cautiously. Our target is generally to keep serum glucose between 140–180 mg/dL avoiding too tight control.

High positive end expiratory pressure (PEEP) can improve oxygenation in patients with sepsis complicated by acute respiratory distress syndrome. High PEEP is not contraindicated in patients with raised intracranial pressure, but the effect of gradual increases in PEEP on the intracranial pressure need to be carefully monitored.

Sedation should be guided by a protocol with a clear goal (e.g., a sedation level defined by the Richmond Agitation Sedation Scale, RASS) and scheduled drug interruptions. These sedation holidays allow us to follow the neurological examination and also reduce the incidence of delirium (see chapter 17). We must remember that opiates are excellent analgesic agents but will greatly confound the neurological examination. The confounding effect of opiates may be quite prolonged in elderly patients and those with liver or renal failure.

Our patient was promptly resuscitated with fluids and norepinephrine. Broad-spectrum antibiotics were started within 30 minutes of the onset of hypotension. The source of sepsis was eventually recognized to be ventilator associated pneumonia. Despite rapid control of the hypotension and adequate treatment of the infection, the brief hypotension proved too much for our patient. He remained stuporous and a repeat head CT scan four days later showed multifocal brain infarctions. This case illustrates that the brain is exquisitely sensitive to ischemia, particularly after a major initial insult such as SAH in our case.

Fever is ubiquitous in critically ill patients and central fever is even more common in patients with acute brain injury. Pancultures should be obtained including CSF when appropriate (meningitis may cause severe sepsis) Yet, when fever is accompanied by hypotension, patients should be rapidly treated for early sepsis following a comprehensive protocol. Any delay in reversing the situation may cause additional brain injury.

### Further Reading

American College of Chest Physicians. Society of Critical Care Medicine Consensus Conference: definitions for sepsis and organ failure and guidelines for the use of innovative therapies in sepsis. *Crit Care Med* 1992; 20:864–874.

Daniels R. Surviving the first hours in sepsis: getting the basics right (an intensivist's perspective). *J Antimicrob Chemother*. 2011;Suppl 2:ii11–ii23.

Dellinger RP, Levy MM, Carlet JM, Bion J, Parker MM, Jaeschke R et al for the International Surviving Sepsis Campaign Guidelines Committee. Surviving Sepsis Campaign: international guidelines for management of severe sepsis and septic shock. *Crit Care Med* 2008; 36:296–327.

Godoy DA, Di Napoli M, Rabinstein AA. Treating hyperglycemia in neurocritical patients: benefits and perils. *Neurocrit Care* 2010; 13:425–438.

National Heart, Lung, and Blood Institute Acute Respiratory Distress Syndrome (ARDS) Clinical Trials Network. Comparison of two fluid management strategies in acute lung injury. *N Engl J Med* 2006; 354:2564–2575.

Rivers E, Nguyen B, Havstad S, Ressler J, Muzzin A, Knoblich B, Peterson E, Tomlanovich M; Early Goal-Directed Therapy Collaborative Group. Early goal-directed therapy in the treatment of severe sepsis and septic shock. *N Engl J Med* 2001; 345:1368–1377.

Russell JA. Management of sepsis. *N Engl J Med* 2006; 355:1699–1713.

# 19 Acute Pulmonary Edema After Major Trauma

A 17-year-old boy traveled with high speed through a dust cloud and had a collision with a truck. According to the first responders he was alert but dazed before he was brought by helicopter to our emergency department. His neurologic examination was completely normal, and he could clearly describe the sequence of events before and after the accident. CT scan of the brain was normal. He was in severe pain in his left leg and was found to have a significantly displaced femoral fracture. He was admitted to the orthopedic ward after undergoing fixation. He asked for opioids frequently to control his pain but remained alert and oriented. Three days after the operation, he suddenly developed respiratory distress and very shortly thereafter he became comatose with irregular breathing. His neurologic examination reveals small reactive pupils, intact corneal reflexes, but extensor motor responses. CT scan of the brain is unchanged, but the X-ray of the chest reveals diffuse infiltrates ("white-out" lungs) (Figure 19.1). He is emergently intubated and transferred to the surgical intensive care unit. You are asked for an opinion on his neurologic examination and whether this represents "neurogenic" pulmonary edema.

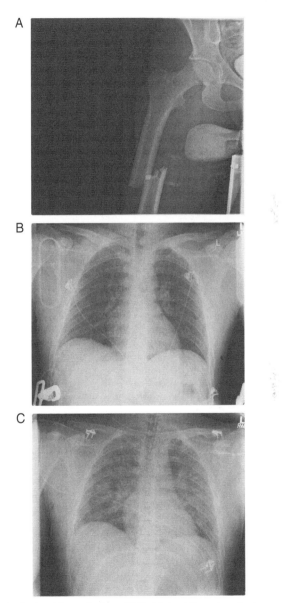

**FIGURE 19.1** Note displaced femur fracture. (A) Serial chest X-rays in patient example: B) normal on admission and C) diffuse pulmonary edema 12 hours later.

Acute pulmonary distress in a patient after significant trauma has multiple causes. In the acute setting, several disorders should be considered, and they include pulmonary contusion, aspiration pneumonitis, and the much less common neurogenic pulmonary edema. Pulmonary emboli are usually seen after a considerable time interval, but they may occur after only a few days of immobilization in predisposed patients. In these patients X-ray is normal but there is a significant hypoxemia not improving with incremental oxygen administration (refractory A-a gradient) because of a large ventilation-perfusion mismatch. A pulmonary embolus should always be considered after neurosurgical procedures, prolonged bed rest, and in patients with hemiplegia in whom the paralyzed leg is particularly at risk of developing deep venous thrombosis. Helical CT angiogram of the chest has become the standard diagnostic test. Acute respiratory distress in a mechanically ventilated patient may have multiple other causes, including acute main bronchus obstruction, inappropriate ventilator settings, pneumothorax, atelectasis, or dislodgement of the tracheostomy tube.

Flash pulmonary edema in a patient with an acute traumatic brain injury is another concerning situation that immediately will lead to intubation and need for high positive end expiratory pressures (PEEP) to open up the collapsed and filled alveoli. The effects of high PEEP on intracranial pressure need to be carefully monitored in patients with head trauma. In hemodynamically unstable patients, high PEEP may reduce cardiac venous return and lead to worsening hypotension. Flash pulmonary edema is usually a result of increased sympathetic activation due to an acute medulla oblongata lesion or due to a rapidly increased intracranial pressure. Pulmonary arterial constriction leads to shunting to other areas that cannot handle pressure, resulting in capillary leak and edema. It can also be seen as a secondary phenomenon of severe stress-induced cardiomyopathy (takotsubo cardiomyopathy). In these patients, there is significant apical ballooning from a major sympathetic outburst associated with acute brain injury, in turn resulting in severe pulmonary edema. Vasodilators and diuretics may be used to relieve pulmonary congestion and reduce ventricular preload. A stress induced cardiomyopathy requires specific treatment to improve ventricular contractility. Fortunately, surviving patients recover quite quickly with a good prognosis.

On paper, this case can be recognized as a classic presentation of fat embolism syndrome. Acute coma and respiratory distress in a patient with a recent femur fracture are sufficient clues to arrive at the diagnosis. In practice, this entity is not always so easily recognized, and reports are infrequently published. Furthermore, the diagnosis is difficult to prove; the "textbook" truncal and axillary petechiae may disappear quickly, fat in bronchial secretions suctioned out by bronchoscopy and fat globules in urine may not be found. (Identification of fat globules requires a special stain such as Sudan red, which is often not readily available.)

Fat embolization syndrome is rare but can be recognized usually about 48 hours after trauma. The treatment of fat embolization syndrome remains supportive and requires hemodynamic stabilization and adequate oxygenation and ventilation with PEEP. Oxygenation goal should be at least an arterial PO2 more than 60 mmHg. Ventilation should maintain plateau pressure less than 30 cm of water and low tidal volumes (6 ml/kg of ideal body weight) to prevent volutrauma.

Fat emboli to the brain may be a cause of sudden neurologic deterioration from injury to the gray and white matter, which may be severe enough to produce coma. Patients may remain comatose for weeks but then may slowly awaken and go on to recover. MRI abnormalities can be particularly severe with numerous lesions reminiscent of a "star field," and often this has been incorrectly interpreted as an indicator of poor outcome.

Our patient recovered very well with supportive care, and the MRI findings disappeared. This case also taught us that fat emboli to the brain resulting in coma (even with motor extensor responses and episodes of paroxysmal hyperactivity) may have a good outcome against all odds.

All these conditions are not common and we should expect more mundaine causes in a trauma patient who develops sudden respiratory distress. Most patients with decreased level of consciousness cannot handle oral secretions, and a weak cough with pooling will lead to bronchial obstruction. Intubation is needed and bronchoscopy will be most helpful in these cases. Neurogenic pulmonary edema is just as rare as fat embolization syndrome. More likely, patients either develop an aspiration pneumonitis

TABLE 19.1 **Acute Pulmonary Conditions after Brain Injury**

| | Neurogenic Pulmonary Edema | Aspiration | Fat Emboli | Pulmonary Embolus |
|---|---|---|---|---|
| *Onset* | Hyperacute | < 6hr | Delayed | Delayed |
| *Clues* | SAH, acute brainstem injury | Intubation, vomiting, seizure | Long bone fracture | Bed rest, fever |
| *Chest X-ray* | Flash edema | Lobar/ multilobar | Flash edema in most severe cases | Normal |
| *Therapy* | PEEP | Broad spectrum antibiotics | PEEP | Anticoagulation, IVC filter, thrombolysis |

SAH, subarachnoid hemorrhage; PEEP, positive end expiratory pressure; IVC, inferior vena cava.

evolving into ARDS or have pulmonary emboli. Both conditions have quite distinctive features that can be distinguished on chest X-ray and CT of the chest. Treatments are specific to those disorders. The differences between pulmonary complications in acute brain injury are shown in Table 19.1.

**KEY POINTS TO REMEMBER REGARDING ACUTE PULMONARY EDEMA AFTER MAJOR TRAUMA**

- Acute pulmonary edema after trauma may be due to cardiogenic or neurogenic pulmonary edema, but the pure forms are infrequent. Aspiration is more common, particularly after a seizure, vomiting, and difficult intubation.
- Clinical suspicion of acute pulmonary emboli is based on sudden oxygen desaturation with increased A-a gradient, but normal X-chest.
- Consider fat emboli in a patient with a recent major long bone fracture who develops sudden respiratory failure and neurological decline.
- Treatment may include broad spectrum antibiotics (suspected aspiration), high PEEP (flash pulmonary edema), and repeated bronchoscopy.

## Further Reading

Akhtar S. Fat embolism. *Anesthesiol Clin.* 2009; 27:533–50,

Bahloul M, Chaari AN, Kallel H, et al. Neurogenic pulmonary edema due to traumatic brain injury: evidence of cardiac dysfunction. *Am J Crit Care* 2006;15:462–470.

Baumann A, Audibert G, McDonnell J, Mertes PM. Neurogenic pulmonary edema. *Acta Anaesthesiol Scand* 2007;51:447–455.

Fontes RBV, Aguiar PH, Zanetti MV, Andrade F, Mandel M, Teixeira MJ. Acute neurogenic pulmonary edema: case reports and literature review. *J Neurosurg Anesth* 2003; 15:144–150.

Habashi NM, Andrews PL, Scalea TM. Therapeutic aspects of fat embolism syndrome. *Injury* 2006; 37:S68–73.

Matthay MA, Zemans RL. The acute respiratory distress syndrome: pathogenesis and treatment. *Annu Rev Pathol.* 2011: 6:147–63.

Rimoldi S, Yuzefpolskaya M, Allemann Y, Messerli F. Flash pulmonary edema. *Cardiovasc Dis* 2009; 52:249–259.

Ware LB, Matthay MA. The acute respiratory distress syndrome. *N Engl J Med* 2000; 342:1334–1349.

# Paroxysmal Sympathetic Hyperactivity

A 22-year-old woman rolled over with her car while driving unrestrained on an icy road. She was comatose at the scene, and she was intubated. Initial head CT scan revealed bifrontal contusions and a small subdural hematoma overlying the right cerebral convexity without significant mass effect. She remained comatose with extensor posturing. An intraparenchymal pressure monitor was inserted. Over the subsequent days the intracranial pressures ranged mostly between 15 and 25 mmHg, requiring occasional doses of 20% mannitol and 10% hypertonic saline to keep it under control. Repeat head CT scan on day three showed the expected evolution of the frontal contusions with progression of the surrounding edema.

Seven days after the injury she starts to exhibit recurrent episodes of sinus tachycardia, tachypnea, hypertension, profuse sweating, and extensor posturing, She is also hyperthermic during the episodes. They are not associated with major episodes of oxygen desaturation, and arterial blood gases do not reveal hypoxia. Blood cultures are negative, and serum lactic acid and creatine kinase levels are normal. Electroencephalogram does not demonstrate epileptiform activity during the spells. When severe, these episodes are associated with transient elevations of intracranial pressure beginning after the onset of the changes in vital signs.

**What do you do now?**

The clinical presentation illustrated by this case is characteristic of paroxysmal sympathetic hyperactivity (PSH). All too frequently PSH remains unrecognized and goes untreated. Physicians who are unfamiliar with this complication may consider these manifestations a mere epiphenomenon of severe brain injury, may obsessively focus on searching for an infectious source or, worse, treat it as seizures with multiple doses of benzodiazepines. PSH can cause major problems in itself. In comatose patients with reduced intracranial compliance, PSH episodes can produce marked rises in intracranial pressure. Also, when PSH is not adequately treated, the severity of the dystonia can result in contractures and make later rehabilitation efforts difficult.

These spells, also known as "sympathetic storms" (or with the misnomer "diencephalic seizures"), are relatively frequent in patients with severe acute brain injury. They are most common in young patients with diffuse axonal traumatic brain injury, but we have also seen them after severe anoxic-ischemic encephalopathy, large intraparenchymal hemorrhages, subarachnoid hemorrhage, and acute hydrocephalus. Episodes of PSH can begin during the acute phase, often in comatose patients. PSH can also continue into the subacute phase or become first manifest in this later phase and diagnosed by brain rehabilitation specialists.

There is lack of uniformity in the nomenclature and definition of PSH. The denomination PSH includes the three terms that describe the main features. They are rapid and episodic (i.e., paroxysmal) manifestations of excessive sympathetic activity. Patients become tachycardic, hypertensive (with increased pulse pressure), tachypneic, febrile, diaphoretic, and often they develop markedly increased muscle tone, which may result in dystonic postures. Pupillary dilatation, piloerection, and skin flushing can also be seen. Spells of PSH are often provoked by stimulation, but the degree of stimulation necessary to trigger the spells can be minimal in the most sensitive patients, and episodes can also occur without apparent provocation.

Proposed diagnostic criteria for severe episodes of PSH are shown in Table 20.1.

The spells are typical and the diagnosis should be readily apparent to the experienced examiner. However, it is always prudent to consider other causes of sudden, exaggerated sympathetic response. Pulmonary embolism and early sepsis with bacteriemia should come to mind. However, pulmonary

TABLE 20.1 **Diagnostic Criteria for Paroxysmal Sympathetic Hyperactivity**

| Clinical Feature | Diagnostic parameter |
| --- | --- |
| Tachycardia | Greater than 140 beats per minute |
| Hypertension | SBP greater than 160 mmHg |
| Fever | Greater than 39 degrees Celsius |
| Tachypnea | Greater than 30 breaths per minute |
| Diaphoresis | Markedly increased |
| Dystonic posturing | Present |

SBP, systolic blood pressure

embolism is distinctly associated with hypoxia and increased alveolar-arterial oxygen gradient, unlike PSH. Meanwhile, sepsis does not present with hypertension, as PSH does. Other pertinent differential diagnoses are listed in Table 20.2.

There are effective therapies for this condition (Table 20.3) and there are also drugs that should be avoided as they can exacerbate the problem. Acutely, the manifestations of PSH respond best to bolus doses of morphine sulfate (2–8 mg intravenously). This favorable response is not related to the analgesic effect of opiates, but rather to modulation of central pathways responsible for the autonomic dysfunction. The response to morphine is rapid and quite reliable in aborting spells of PSH, but occasionally we have encountered patients who required much larger doses than usual (up to 10–15 mg). In these patients a continuous opiate infusion may be helpful.

Other effective medications for the treatment of PSH include noncardioselective beta-blockers (such as propranolol), clonidine (a central alpha 2-receptor agonist), dexmedetomidine (another central alpha 2 receptor agonist), bromocriptine (a dopamine D2-receptor agonist), baclofen (a $GABA_B$ receptor agonist), benzodiazepines ($GABA_A$ receptor agonist), and gabapentin (which binds GABA receptors and voltage-gated calcium channels in the dorsal horn of the spinal cord). In our experience, beta-blockers and clonidine are useful in controlling the tachycardia and hypertension, but less so for the dystonia. Baclofen and benzodiazepines (especially diazepam) do cause muscle relaxation, but may not improve the other

| To rule out | You should check |
| --- | --- |
| Pulmonary embolism | Arterial blood gases<br>CT angiogram of the chest |
| Sepsis* | White blood cell count<br>Blood cultures<br>Serum lactic acid |
| Seizures | Electroencephalogram |
| Neuroleptic malignant syndrome | History of neuroleptic exposure<br>Serum creatine kinase<br>Response to dantrolene |
| Serotonin syndrome | History of use of proserotonin drugs<br>Serum creatine kinase<br>Response to cyproheptadine |
| Alcohol withdrawal | History of alcohol abuse<br>Response to benzodiazepines |
| Cushing response | Brain imaging |
| Autonomic dysreflexia from spinal cord injury** | Spinal cord imaging |
| Encephalitis | Cerebrospinal fluid |
| Aneurysmal rebleeding in subarachnoid hemorrhage | Repeat brain imaging |

*Typically associated with hypotension rather than hypertension
**Typically associated with bradycardia rather than tachycardia

hypersympathetic features. We have seen dramatic improvement in the frequency and severity of spells within days of starting gabapentin, which has become our first choice for the longer-term control of this disorder. We have not been impressed by the efficacy of bromocriptine. Antidopaminergic drugs, such as haloperidol, and sympathetic agonists need to be avoided.

Choosing the right medication to treat the spells is not enough, and other aspects of management are equally important. These patients sweat profusely and fluid intake should be adjusted to compensate for this marked

TABLE 20.3 **Pharmacological Options for the Treatment of Paroxysmal Sympathetic Hyperactivity**

| Medication | Usual Dose | Usefulness | Side Effects |
|---|---|---|---|
| Morphine sulfate | 2–8 mg IV bolus | Abortive | Sedation<br>Respiratory depression<br>Hypotension<br>Ileus<br>Raised ICP (rare) |
| Propranolol | 20–60 mg every 4–8 hrs by enteral route | Preventive control of tachycardia and hypertension | Bradycardia<br>Hypotension<br>Bronchospasm<br>Negative inotropism |
| Clonidine | 0.1–0.3 mg every 6–8 hrs by enteral route | Preventive control of tachycardia and hypertension | Bradycardia<br>Hypotension<br>Sedation<br>Rebound hypertension with abrupt withdrawal |
| Dexmedetomidine | 0.2–0.7 mcg/kg/hr | Preventive | Bradycardia<br>Hypotension<br>Sedation |
| Baclofen | 5–10 mg every 8 hrs (up to 60–80 mg/day) by enteral route* | Control of increased muscle tone | Sedation<br>Increased muscle weakness<br>Hepatotoxicity<br>Increased respiratory secretions |
| Diazepam | 50–10 mg IV every 4–8 hrs | Control of increased muscle tone | Sedation<br>Hypotension<br>Respiratory depression |
| Gabapentin | Start 300 mg every 8 hrs by enteral route and titrate up to 1,800–3,600 mg/day | Preventive | Mild sedation |

ICP, intracranial pressure; IV intravenous
*Intrathecal baclofen can be useful in refractory cases with extreme dystonia.

increase in insensible losses and to prevent volume contraction. Fever must be aggressively treated with cooling measures as it has a negative impact on the acutely injured brain. It is best to minimize patient stimulation.

How did we manage our patient? We treated her acutely with boluses of morphine, and she responded well. Her tachycardia and hypertension improved on low doses of propranolol. We also started her on gabapentin with a target dose of 1,800 mg per day. Ten days later her episodes of PSH had become much milder and infrequent and they were no longer manifested with dystonia.

PSH is often associated with poor neurologic outcome but not invariably so. The manifestations excessively increase the metabolic demand, risk increase in intracranial pressure, and may cause long-term complications. Because it is a relatively common and treatable complication in comatose patients, physicians need to be aware of it and be prepared to initiate effective therapy.

---

### KEY POINTS TO REMEMBER REGARDING PAROXYSMAL SYMPATHETIC HYPERACTIVITY (PSH)

- PSH is not uncommon, especially in young patients with severe traumatic brain injury.
- The differential diagnosis is broad, but can be sorted out quickly by a focused evaluation. When the clinical signs are not characteristic consider pulmonary embolism, early sepsis, and seizures.
- Lack of recognition of PSH can lead to major complications, such as intracranial hypertension, dehydration, refractory fever, refractory surges of hypertension, and muscle contractures.
- Boluses of morphine sulfate are effective in aborting the episodes, propranolol and clonidine can help control the tachycardia and hypertension, baclofen and diazepam can improve the increased muscle tone.
- Gabapentin is very useful to achieve control of the sympathetic dysfunction in the long-term.

**Further Reading**

Baguley IJ, Heriseanu RE, Cameron ID, Nott MT, Slewa-Younan S. A critical review of the pathophysiology of dysautonomia following traumatic brain injury. *Neurocrit Care* 2008; 8:293-300.

Baguley IJ, Heriseanu RE, Gurka JA, Nordenbo A, Cameron ID. Gabapentin in the management of dysautonomia following severe traumatic brain injury: a case series. *J Neurol Neurosurg Psychiatry* 2007; 78:539-541.

Blackman JA, Patrick PD, Buck ML, Rust RS Jr. Paroxysmal autonomic instability with dystonia after brain injury. *Arch Neurol* 2004; 61:321-328.

Boeve BF, Wijdicks EF, Benarroch EE, Schmidt KD. Paroxysmal sympathetic storms ("diencephalic seizures") after severe diffuse axonal head injury. *Mayo Clin Proc* 1998; 73:148-152.

Perkes I, Baguley IJ, Nott MT, Menon DK. A review of paroxysmal sympathetic hyperactivity after acquired brain injury. *Ann Neurol* 2010; 68,126-135.

Rabinstein AA. Paroxysmal sympathetic hyperactivity in the neurological intensive care unit. *Neurol Res* 2007; 29:680-682.

Rabinstein AA, Benarroch EE. Treatment of paroxysmal sympathetic hyperactivity. *Curr Treat Options Neurol* 2008; 10:151-157.

# Acute Hypertension After Stroke

A 56-year-old man with history of long-standing poorly controlled hypertension presents to the emergency department with sudden onset of a speech abnormality and right-sided weakness. Time from symptom onset is 70 minutes. First examination reveals a global aphasia, right heminopia, right hemiparesis (NIH stroke scale of 14).

Head CT scan shows a probable hyperdense dot sign in a Sylvian branch of the left middle cerebral artery with no evidence of acute infarction or hemorrhage. Blood pressure is initially 204/112 mmHg. He responds only briefly to two doses of 10 mg of intravenous labetalol each. The patient is potentially a candidate for intravenous thrombolysis, but after these two doses of labetalol, the blood pressure is back up to 194/106 mmHg. There are no other clinical or laboratory contraindications for intravenous thrombolysis.

*What do you do now?*

To know how—or even when—to treat hypertension in a patient with acute stroke, three pieces of information are needed. First, one needs to know the type of stroke, second, the time from the onset of symptoms and third, in acute ischemic stroke whether the patient is a candidate for thrombolysis (Figure 21.1). All recommendations mentioned here on blood pressure management are based on collective experience of experts in the field but, unfortunately, no clinical trials have evaluated this matter. Several clinical scenarios can be expected in the emergency department or neurosciences intensive care unit (NICU), and they are categorized as follows.

## Ischemic Stroke-Candidate for Thrombolysis–First 24 Hours

Patients who are candidates for thrombolysis need to have their hypertension reliably controlled before they can be treated with rt-PA. Expert guidelines recommend reducing the systolic blood pressure below 185 mmHg and the diastolic blood pressure below 110 mmHg before infusing the

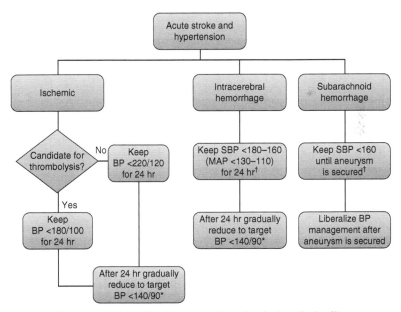

**FIGURE 21.1** Recommended algorithm for control of hypertension in patients with acute stroke. *Target should be 130/80 mmHg in patients with diabetes mellitus. Ideal blood pressure < 120/80 mm Hg. † If suspected increased intracranial pressure, then monitor intracranial pressure and maintain cerebral perfusion pressure > 60 mmHg. BP; blood pressure.

thrombolytic. If these parameters cannot be reached and consistently maintained, intravenous rt-PA should not be administered. The same principle applies to endovascular recanalization therapies (mechanical clot retrieval or suctioning, intracranial stent placement). The rationale for deferring any type of acute recanalization therapies in patients with uncontrolled hypertension is that the risk of reperfusion hemorrhage is likely too high.

Following thrombolysis (or acute endovascular therapy), the blood pressure should be monitored closely (every 15 minutes for the first 2–3 hours, then every 30 minutes for 6 hours, and then hourly for the rest of the first day), and kept below 180/105 mmHg. Failure to control hypertension during this first day could result in a cerebral hematoma with rapid neurologic deterioration.

In our patient, we were able to reduce the blood pressure to an acceptable range after initiating an infusion of nicardipine, which was then continued for 24 hours in the NICU. The patient received intravenous rt-PA and improved substantially over the following day. On the second hospital day we restarted his ACE inhibitor and started a thiazide. Later the dose of the ACE inhibitor was progressively adjusted until blood pressure was normalized. His discharge NIH stroke scale was 3 and he only had minor symptoms and no disability 3 months later.

### Ischemic Stroke–Not Candidate for Thrombolysis–First 24 Hours

Hypertension may be a physiological response in patients with acute brain ischemia (as indicated by the spontaneous resolution of hypertension typically seen after successful recanalization). Therefore, when the patient is not a candidate for acute recanalization therapy the prevailing thought is that it is better not to lower the blood pressure unless it is exceedingly high (above 220/120 mmHg). The concept of accepting high blood pressures ("permissive hypertension") is based on the notion that lowering the blood pressure in these patients with persistent vessel occlusion could worsen the brain ischemia by reducing collateral flow. When allowing blood pressure to remain high, it is important to monitor patients for possible signs of congestive heart failure, acute kidney injury, and other complications of acute hypertension. That said, gradual and modest blood pressure reduction (by 10 or 15 mmHg) is probably safe, and studies are investigating whether this approach can be beneficial.

## Ischemic Stroke—After the First 24 Hours

After the first day, we gradually start oral medications (beginning with any medications the patient was taking before admission if any had been prescribed) with the purpose of progressively achieving normotension while avoiding sudden drops in blood pressure. If the blood pressure control is not optimal upon discharge, we arrange for very close follow-up as outpatient until the goal of blood pressure normalization is reached.

## Intracerebral Hemorrhage—First 24 Hours

Patients with intracerebral hemorrhage should be treated to achieve moderate blood pressure reduction (systolic blood pressure < 180–160 mmHg, mean arterial pressure < 130–110 mmHg). Although cerebral hematomas are surrounded by an area of hypoperfusion, these areas are not oxygen deprived as is typical of penumbral tissue, and there is no evidence that moderately reducing the blood pressure a few hours after hematoma onset can cause worsening ischemia. Moreover profound hypertension (especially when mean arterial pressure is over 140 mmHg) increases the risk of hematoma expansion. The possible value of more aggressive blood pressure reduction in these patients is currently being evaluated in prospective clinical trials.

We lower the blood pressure of patients with intracerebral hemorrhage starting as soon as the diagnosis is made, but try to do so gradually to avoid compromising cerebral perfusion. If intracranial pressure is monitored, rarely the case in clinical practice, the cerebral perfusion pressure should be maintained above 60 mmHg.

## Intracerebral Hemorrhage—After the First 24 Hours

Similarly to ischemic stroke, after the first 24 hours we typically initiate oral antihypertensives, which are then titrated to achieve progressive normalization of the blood pressure before or shortly following discharge from the hospital.

## Aneurysmal Subarachnoid Hemorrhage

Although there is no good evidence to guide the treatment of hypertension in acute aneurysmal subarachnoid hemorrhage, we prefer to treat hypertension with the goal of maintaining the systolic blood pressure below 160 mmHg before the aneurysm is secured, but we recognize that the evidence that blood pressure above those values is associated with higher risk of aneurysm rebleeding is not strong. Most patients with aneurysmal subarachnoid hemorrhage have elevated blood pressures due to the excessive sympathetic release that immediately follows the aneurysm rupture. Moreover, in these patients intracranial hypertension is common, and most patients with abnormal level of consciousness will need a ventriculostomy. Acutely lowering the blood pressure in patients with intracranial hypertension could compromise cerebral perfusion pressure. When intracranial pressure is known, the cerebral perfusion pressure should be kept above 60 mmHg.

Once the aneurysm is treated by means of clipping or endovascular coiling, we stop antihypertensives except for nimodipine (and low-dose beta-blocker in patients with history of heart disease previously on beta-blockers) anticipating the need to maintain adequate cerebral perfusion in a narrowed arterial bed from vasospasm.

## What Drugs Should You Use?

We prefer labetalol or hydralazine in intermittent doses (both 10 mg IV) and we choose between them depending on the heart rate (if bradycardia, it is safer to use hydralazine). Enalaprilat is another reasonable option. If intermittent doses of these medications fail to control the hypertension, we place an arterial catheter and start an infusion of nicardipine (or sometimes labetalol). Clevidipine, a newer dihydropyridine calcium channel blocker, also appears to be a safe and effective agent for the acute control of severe hypertension. The most severe and refractory cases of acute hypertension may necessitate treatment with sodium nitroprusside. We prefer to avoid nitrates because their known venodilatory effect can increase intracranial pressure, although we are not so certain about the claimed deleterious effect on intracranial pressure with sodium nitroprusside. We also avoid very rapidly acting medications, such as sublingual nifedipine, because they can provoke excessive drops in blood pressure. Clonidine is not a safe option either in the hyperacute phase because the first dose can occasionally cause paradoxical hypertension. Table 21.1 lists the doses of the medications we use most often for the treatment of acute hypertension in ischemic and hemorrhagic stroke.

TABLE 21.1 **Options for the Treatment of Hypertension in Patients with Acute Stroke**

| Drug | Usual dose |
|---|---|
| Labetalol | 10-20 mg IV over 1-2 minutes, may repeat after 10-15 minutes (maximum dose 300 mg over 24 hours) <br> Infusion: 2-8 mg/min |
| Hydralazine | 10-20 mg IV over 1-2 minutes, may repeat after 10-15 minutes |
| Nicardipine | Infusion: 5 mg/hr, then can be titrated up to 15 mg/hr as needed |
| Sodium nitroprusside | Infusion: 0.3 mcg/kg/min, then can be titrated up to 10 mcg/kg/min as needed |

**KEY POINTS TO REMEMBER REGARDING ACUTE HYPERTENSION AFTER STROKE**

- The goals of treatment of hypertension in acute stroke patients depends on the type of stroke and the time from symptom onset.
- Ischemic stroke patients receiving thrombolysis need strict and consistent control of hypertension to avoid hemorrhagic complications.
- Patients with ischemic stroke who are not candidates for recanalization therapies should have their hypertension managed more conservatively to avoid decrease in collateral cerebral blood flow.
- In patients with acute intracerebral hemorrhage moderate reductions of blood pressure are safe and may reduce the chances of hematoma expansion.
- In aneurysmal subarachnoid hemorrhage, we favor gradual blood pressure reduction during the first few hours which we maintain until the aneurysm is treated. Then blood pressure parameters should change upward to reduce the risk of ischemia if cerebral vasospasm develops.

## Further Reading

Adams HP Jr, del Zoppo G, Alberts MJ, Bhatt DL, Brass L, Furlan A, Grubb RL, Higashida RT, Jauch EC, Kidwell C, Lyden PD, Morgenstern LB, Qureshi AI, Rosenwasser RH, Scott PA, Wijdicks EF; American Heart Association; American Stroke Association Stroke Council; Clinical Cardiology Council; Cardiovascular Radiology and Intervention Council; Atherosclerotic Peripheral Vascular Disease and Quality of Care Outcomes in Research Interdisciplinary Working Groups. Guidelines for the early management of adults with ischemic stroke: a guideline from the American Heart Association/American Stroke Association Stroke Council, Clinical Cardiology Council, Cardiovascular Radiology and Intervention Council, and the Atherosclerotic Peripheral Vascular Disease and Quality of Care Outcomes in Research Interdisciplinary Working Groups: the American Academy of Neurology affirms the value of this guideline as an educational tool for neurologists. *Stroke* 2007; 38:1655-1711.

Aiyagari V, Gorelick PB. Management of blood pressure for acute and recurrent stroke. *Stroke* 2009;40:2251-2256.

Anderson CS, Huang Y, Want JG, et al. Intensive blood pressure reduction in acute cerebral hemorrhage trial (INTERACT): a randomized pilot trial. *Lancet Neurol* 2008;7:391-399.

Geeganage C, Bath PM. Vasoactive drugs for acute stroke *Cochrane Database Syst Rev.* 2010; 7:CD002839.

Katzan IL, Furlan AJ, Lloyd LE, Frank JI, Harper DL, Hinchey JA, Hammel JP, Qu A, Sila CA. Use of tissue-type plasminogen activator for acute ischemic stroke: the Cleveland area experience. *JAMA* 2000; 283:1151-1158.

Marik PE, Varon J. Hypertensive crises, challenges and management. *Chest* 2007;131:1949-1962.

Morgenstern LB, Hemphill JC 3rd, Anderson C, Becker K, Broderick JP, Connolly ES Jr, Greenberg SM, Huang JN, MacDonald RL, Messé SR, Mitchell PH, Selim M, Tamargo RJ; American Heart Association Stroke Council and Council on Cardiovascular Nursing. Guidelines for the management of spontaneous intracerebral hemorrhage: a guideline for healthcare professionals from the American Heart Association/American Stroke Association. *Stroke* 2010; 41:2108-2129.

Potter JF, Robinson TG, Ford GA, Mistri A, James M, Chernova J, Jagger C. Controlling hypertension and hypotension immediately post-stroke (CHHIPS): a randomized, placebo-controlled, double-blind pilot trial. *Lancet Neurol.* 2009; 8:48-56.

Rabinstein AA, Lanzino G, Wijdicks EFM. Multidisciplinary management and emerging therapeutic strategies in aneurysmal subarachnoid hemorrhage. *Lancet Neurol* 2010; 9:504-519.

Stead LG, Gilmore RM, Vedula KC, Weaver AL, Decker WW, Brown RD Jr. Impact of acute blood pressure variability on ischemic stroke outcome. *Neurology* 2006; 66:1878-1881.

# Acute Cardiac Arrhythmia After Acute Brain Injury

An 86-year-old patient with a prior history of hypertension, hyperlipidemia, and atrial fibrillation presents with difficulty speaking and right-sided numbness. On examination, she has apraxia of speech and right hemiparesis. An MRI shows a left internal carotid occlusion with acute ischemic change in the left cerebral hemisphere. Systolic blood pressure is fluctuating and at times 130 mmHg. It appears that her speech problems also fluctuate, and a possible link between worsening aphasia and relative hypotension is assumed. The decision is made to discontinue atenolol to maintain a higher blood pressure. Within 12 hours, the patient develops a rapid ventricular response to her atrial fibrillation with a pulse up to 140 beats per minute. Serum troponin has increased to 0.16 ng/ml. The electrocardiogram (EKG) shows rate-related repolarization changes (Figure 22.1). The patient is transferred to the Neurosciences Intensive Care Unit for acute management.

**What do you do now?**

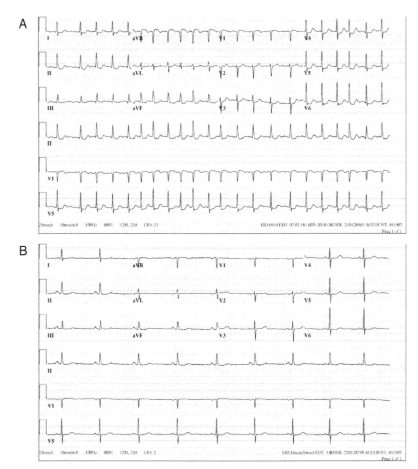

**FIGURE 22.1** EKG: Atrial fibrillation and rapid ventricular response (A) with resolution (B).

Cardiac arrhythmias and EKG changes are quite common in patients with critical neurologic illness, often need more than cursory attention and management may become complex. Cardiac arrhythmias are often brief periods of premature beats, sinus bradycardia, or, as it is in our case, atrial fibrillation with rapid ventricular response. Conversely, an intracerebral hematoma may coincide with long-standing atrial fibrillation. An intracranial hemorrhage can be an unintended consequence of warfarin therapy to protect the patient from an ischemic stroke. In patients with an ischemic stroke, atrial fibrillation may not have been treated with warfarin or may have been recently discontinued for a surgical procedure leading to mobilization of an atrial thrombus to a major cerebral artery. In other patients there may be no direct correlation, and a carotid or basilar artery occludes from progressive atherosclerotic disease, such as in our patient example.

After an acute ischemic stroke patients may have a relatively low to normal blood pressure, and that is partly due to sudden bed rest and relative dehydration. "Low" systolic blood pressure (less than 155 mmHg) has been associated with increased mortality after a stroke, but the nature of the relationship remains unexplained. This all provides a motivation to increase the blood pressure in the acute stage. Not infrequently, beta-blockers are first discontinued to allow for higher blood-pressures. This may provide better perfusion in collaterals and could reduce the ischemic area.

However, the risks of such an intervention are not known. Stopping rate control medication in patients with atrial fibrillation may result in tachycardia that could lead to demand ischemia, which may be more severe in patients with coronary artery disease. This occurred in our case example with an increase in serum troponin.

The treatment for atrial fibrillation with rapid ventricular rate is either calcium channel blockers (for example intravenous diltiazem) beta-blockers, or amiodarone. These drugs control ventricular rate successfully, but amiodarone induces less hypotension and has higher frequency of converting patients with new onset atrial fibrillation into normal sinus rhythm. Cardioversion is rarely attempted in acute stroke because 1) patients often would need at least two days of anticoagulation, 2) hypotension might be deleterious to the patient, and 3) atrial fibrillation is often long-standing and patients are unlikely to stay in sinus rhythm. After control of the ventricular response is achieved, oral doses of beta-blockers (i.e. metoprolol) are administered to maintain rate control.

It is true that cardiac arrhythmias are prevalent in the NICU, but they may just be transient and without any consequence. Drug induced arrhythmias should be excluded. However, any new cardiac arrhythmia could point toward new onset sepsis, pulmonary emboli, or sudden blood loss. Acute myocardial ischemia with new cardiac arrhythmias may occur in any patient with a recent neurosurgical procedure. There are far more details that need to be known, but a general guideline for treatment of cardiac arrhythmias is shown in Table 22.1.

Another commonly asked question is whether the EKG changes are a result of the acute neurologic injury (a favorite cardiologist explanation). Morphological EKG changes are common in traumatic brain injury and subarachnoid hemorrhage (typically S-T segment sagging, prolonged QT interval, and symmetrically peaked T-waves often referred to as cerebral T-waves), and patients with ischemic strokes affecting the insula appear to be more prone to cardiac arrhythmias. However, most often it is not prudent to solely attribute cardiac rhythm changes to the acute brain injury. Further cardiac evaluation is necessary in the vast majority of patients.

TABLE 22.1  **Guidance for the Treatment of Common Cardiac Arrhythmias**

| Arrhythmia | Therapy |
| --- | --- |
| Sinus tachycardia | Fluids, esmolol |
| Sinus bradycardia | Atropine, cardiac pacing |
| Atrial fibrillation | Diltiazem, esmolol, amiodarone |
| Multifocal atrial tachycardia | Verapamil or metoprolol |
| Atrioventricular block | Cardiac pacing |
| Ventricular tachycardia | Cardioversion |
| Torsades de pointes | Magnesium sulfate |

Adapted from Wijdicks EFM, *The Practice of Emergency and Critical Care Neurology*, Oxford University Press, New York, 2010.

**Further Reading**

Barnes BJ, Hollands JM. Drug-induced arrhythmias. *Crit Care Med* 2010; 38: S188-197.

Bossone E, DiGiovine B, Watts S et al. Range and prevalence of cardiac abnormalities in patients hospitalized in a Medical ICU. *Chest* 2002; 122:1370-1376.

Goodman S, Weiss Y, Weissman C. Update on cardiac arrhythmias in the ICU. *Curr Opin Crit Care* 2008; 14:549-554.

Oppenheimer S. Cerebrogenic cardiac arrhythmias: Cortical lateralization and clinical significance. *Clin Auton Res* 2006; 16:6-11.

Samuels MA. The brain-heart connection. *Circulation* 2007; 116:77-84.

# 23 Autonomic Failure in Guillain-Barré Syndrome

A 73-year-old man was admitted with progressive weakness and inability to stand unassisted. This was noticed three weeks after a mundane respiratory infection that was briefly treated with antibiotics. The patient started with tingling in all of his extremities followed a day later by rapid onset of weakness for 4 days. Initially, he had no swallowing difficulties, double vision, or shortness of breath; but he was more short-winded and could not swallow liquids well.

On admission, he had a flaccid quadriplegia with generalized areflexia, but also had marked tachypnea that required intubation and mechanical ventilation. On examination, there is a marked bifacial diplegia with limited eye movements. Pupils are sluggish in light responsiveness. He is not overbreathing the ventilator and has a weak cough with tracheal suctioning. There is a flaccid quadriplegia with absent reflexes throughout. The patient is started on intravenous immunoglobulin but, on the fourth day after admission, he starts to develop marked blood pressure fluctuations, and an arterial line is placed. At some point, his systolic blood pressure is measured at 240 mmHg and then suddenly drops to 70 mmHg, which requires a Trendelenburg position. During the following days, these blood pressure fluctuations remain, often with episodes of hypertensive surges. The nursing staff is quite concerned with these readings and would like to have more strict orders and blood pressure goals.

## What do you do now?

The management of a patient with a severe Guillain-Barré syndrome (GBS) is not straightforward. It is not just providing intravenous immunoglobulin or plasma exchange, but also adequate supportive ICU care. Any physician should anticipate that patients with GBS are rapidly at risk for ventilator-associated pneumonia, urinary tract infection and sepsis, decubitus ulcers, and gastrointestinal hemorrhages due to the stress of mechanical ventilation. Deep venous thrombosis will need to be aggressively prevented with intermittent pneumatic compression devices plus subcutaneous heparin injections (Table 23.1).

The most concerning part of management is the treatment of acute autonomic failure, usually observed in the more severe cases. Dysautonomia in GBS is manifested by blood pressure fluctuations, cardiac arrhythmias, bladder dysfunction, gastrointestinal dysfunction, bronchial smooth muscle

TABLE 23.1 **Early Management of Guillain-Barré Syndrome**

IVIG (0.4 g/kg for 5 consecutive days)*

PLEX (5 plasma volumes in 10 days)*

Prevent early complications

　　Subcutaneous heparin 5,000 U 3 x day

　　PPI for GI protection

　　Decubitus protection (special beds)

　　NG tube feeding, consider early PEG in intubated patients, watch for ileus

　　Tracheostomy in severely affected patients

Blood pressure fluctuation and cardiac arrhythmias

　　Low doses of IV morphine.

　　Labetalol, clonidine, or nicardipine

　　Avoid bradycardia with suctioning

　　Consider pacemaker

---

* One course of treatment is typical. Using combinations (PLEX after IVIG or IVIG after PLEX) has not been proven to change outcome, but we have anecdotal experience of improvement with such a combination. A second course of IVIG can also be considered.

PLEX = Plasma exchange; IVIG = intravenous immunoglobulin; PPI = proton pump inhibitors; PEG = percutaneous gastrostomy; GI = gastrointestinal; NG = nasogastric.

dysfunction, and exaggerated drug responses. Most commonly, as exemplified by our patient, the issue at hand is treatment of blood pressure fluctuations. Paroxysmal or sustained hypertension is seen in about one in four patients with a rapid onset of GBS. Systolic blood pressures can become substantially elevated and reach values that could not only challenge ventricular function, but could even predispose the patient to develop posterior reversible encephalopathy syndrome. (Unexpected new onset seizures or marked visual disturbances in a patient with GBS should prompt an MRI scan to look for its characteristic vasogenic edema.)

Why these blood pressure fluctuations occur is not entirely known, but a baroreflex abnormality has been postulated. Baroreceptor sensitivity might be altered as a result of vagal nerve demyelination and because sympathetic nerves have less myelin, there is a sympathetic overdrive. Dysfunction of afferent input from atrial stretch receptors could also play a role in the origin of these blood pressure surges.

These blood pressure elevations would require treatment, but another concern is that treatment might lead to a marked hypotension. This could be due to exaggerated drug sensitivity in GBS, but this phenomenon, although well known, is not adequately understood. Drugs such as clonidine, sodium nitroprusside, or a calcium channel blocker such as nicardipine may be helpful to treat severe hypertension, but in our experience, simply controlling these responses with multiple doses of IV morphine is just as effective and perhaps safer with less hypotension.

Many patients with GBS have a baseline sinus tachycardia as another manifestation of increased sympathetic output. In addition, patients may develop so-called vagal spells, typically after tracheal suctioning. These bradycardic spells may be so severe that they can lead to a brief asystole. A pacemaker may be considered if these episodes are symptomatic and recurrent. In some patients, atrioventricular block or other more benign arrhythmias (e.g., bigeminy) become apparent.

Bronchial function is also likely impaired in Guillain-Barré syndrome, because bronchoconstriction and bronchodilatation are under the control of vagal and sympathetic innervation. There is some evidence that impaired bronchoconstriction and dilation due to abnormal innervation of bronchial smooth muscle can lead to profound impairment of clearing of secretions and, in turn, lead to atelectasis of large lung segments.

As part of the screening for dysautonomia, patients should also be carefully examined for development of adynamic ileus. This occurs in about 1 in 10 patients with severe Guillain-Barré syndrome and is recognized by loss of abdominal sounds, expansion of the abdominal girth, and clearly demonstrable enlarged colonic loops on abdominal x-ray (Figure 23.1). Perforation of the colon is a very concerning complication which can

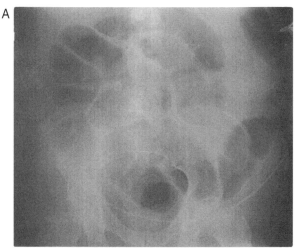

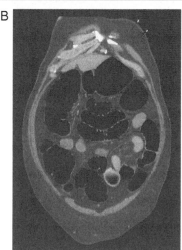

**FIGURE 23.1** Marked dilated colonic loops on abdominal X-ray (A) and confirmed on abdominal CT scan (B).

substantially change the outcome of a recoverable neurologic illness, and can even lead to in-hospital death.

The treatment of patients with adynamic ileus is mostly parenteral nutrition for several weeks, rectal and oral suction tubes, and in more severe cases, a therapeutic decompressive colonoscopy. The use of erythromycin might be considered if patients have gastroparesis, but its side effects (cardiac arrhythmias) in patients with severe dysautonomia may make it a less favorable choice. We discourage the use of metoclopramide as promotility agent, because it has been associated with the occurrence of asystole in GBS.

In our patient, being on a mechanical ventilator made the use of multiple doses of intravenous morphine much safer, and blood pressure could be controlled within the set goal of systolic blood pressures of 100–140 mmHg. The nursing staff was particularly careful with tracheal suctions trying to avoid multiple passages and straining that could lead to bradycardia and hypotension. The blood pressure swings became less apparent in the following weeks with gradual disappearance over time.

Acute autonomic failure in GBS usually resolves before the patient starts to improve motor function. Marked orthostatic hypotension may persist during the recovery phase. Whether this is due to persistent autonomic failure or a result of long-standing bed rest is undetermined.

---

**KEY POINTS TO REMEMBER REGARDING AUTONOMIC FAILURE IN GUILLAIN-BARRÉ SYNDROME**

- Acute autonomic failure is common in severe presentations of GBS. Marked blood pressure fluctuations or sustained hypertension are the most concerning manifestations.
- Hypertensive surges can be treated with morphine, clonidine, or if necessary, an infusion of a calcium channel blocker, such as nicardipine.
- Vagal spells may lead to prolonged episodes of asystole, and a transcutaneous pacemaker might be needed.
- Every bedridden patient with severe GBS is at risk of developing severe adynamic ileus, and treatment may require a period of parenteral nutrition or colonoscopic decompression.

## Further Reading

Cortese I, Chaudry Y, Do YT. Evidence-based guideline update:Plasmapheresis in neurologic disorders:report of the Therapeutics and Technology Assessment Subcommittee of the American Academy of Neurology. *Neurology* 2011;76;294-300.

Hughes RA, Wijdicks EFM, Barohn R, Benson E, Cornblath DR, Hahn AF, Meythaler JM et al. Practice parameter: immunotherapy for Guillain-Barré syndrome: report of the Quality Standards Subcommittee of the American Academy of Neurology. *Neurology* 2003; 61:736-740.

Hughes RA, Wijdicks EFM, Benson E, Cornblath DR, Hahn AF, Meythaler JM, Sladky JT et al. Supportive care for patients with Guillain-Barré syndrome. *Arch Neurol* 2005; 1194-1198.

Mukerji S, Aloka F, Farooq MU, Kassab MY, Abela GS. Cardiovascular complications of the Guillain-Barré syndrome. *Am J Cardiol* 2009; 104:1452-1455.

McDaneld LM, Fields JD, Bourdette DN et al. Immunomodulatory therapies in neurologic critical care. *Neurocrit Care* 2010; 12:132-143.

Van Doorn PA, Ruts L, Jacobs BC. Clinical features, pathogenesis, and treatment of Guillain-Barré syndrome. *Lancet Neurol* 2008; 7:939-950.

# Weaning of the Ventilator in Myasthenia Gravis

A 60-year-old man with a recent diagnosis of myasthenia gravis developed shortness of breath and trouble keeping his head up. In the following days he developed difficulty with swallowing. He was admitted to an outside hospital, where he received three infusions of intravenous immunoglobulin (IVIG), but was found "unresponsive" on the fourth day with an arterial PCO2 greater than 110 mmHg and a pH of 6.8 requiring emergency intubation. He awakened quickly after arterial PCO2 correction, but was found to be profoundly weak. Chest X-ray showed only minor atelectasis. He was transferred to our neurosciences intensive care unit. He was started on oral prednisone and plasma exchange. After 3 exchanges, his muscle strength was significantly better and coughing appeared strong. He was extubated and maintained good oxygenation for several hours; however, during the day, he became increasingly tachypneic and was placed on BiPAP.

His neurologic examination shows good neck flexion, hoarseness, and weak coughing up of secretions. Muscle strength is good in all extremities with no hint of fatigable weakness. However he is barely tolerating BiPAP and is having more trouble with pooling of secretions. Arterial PCO2 climbs to 55 mmHg, and he is reintubated. Chest X-ray shows marked atelectasis of the left lung (Figure 24.1).

**What do you do now?**

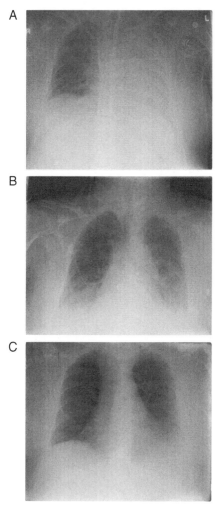

**FIGURE 24.1** Hypersecretion and neuromuscular respiratory failure in myasthenia gravis. Serial X-chest showing marked left atelectasis from a mucus plug (A) and gradual improvement after intubation and bronchoscopy (B, C).

How do you safely get a patient with a recent flare-up of myasthenia gravis off the ventilator and keep him off the ventilator? For one thing, management of myasthenic crisis with neuromuscular respiratory failure remains poorly defined and largely empirical. Quite a few patients will have to be intubated and reintubated. Many do improve rapidly after specific therapy—IVIG, or plasma exchange. A recent analysis concluded that the treatment effects of these two options in myasthenia gravis-and possibly myasthenia crises- are comparable. Delay of treatment however increases mortality and complications.

After neurologic improvement, weaning from the ventilator becomes a priority. Liberating myasthenic patients from the ventilator, however, remains frustrating for most attending physicians. Moreover, pulmonary infections and atelectases can make weaning even more challenging.

Most neurologists will try to find an adequate dose of pyridostigmine that improves muscle strength and oropharyngeal function and could assist in weaning the patient off the ventilator. However, at the same time a dose of pyridostigmine must be found that does not cause abundant secretions. Thick secretions will predispose the patient to sudden mucus plugs, which, as it was in our case, may occlude a large bronchial branch.

There are some prerequisites to consider for physicians attempting to wean the patient from the ventilator. The first priority remains satisfactory treatment of the myasthenic symptoms. This is best accomplished with plasma exchange in the acute phase. In our experience, once the patient is severely affected and intubated, IVIG less frequently will lead to substantial improvement. Multiple bronchoscopies may be necessary to clear the bronchial tree from secretions, and often an infection becomes apparent that requires specific antibiotic treatment. Only after the secretions and infection are under control can the patient be considered for weaning. In some instances, early tracheostomy is necessary to better clear secretions from the airways.

Treatment with immunosuppressive drugs should be started, and usually this includes prednisone 60 to 90 mg and perhaps a pulse-dose of methylprednisolone (intravenous infusion of 1 gram). Long-term treatment with mycophenolate mofetil, for example, will only take effect several weeks after initiation and cannot be relied on in the acute phase of management.

The prediction of success of extubation is difficult to determine clinically, and we have not found a good way to do it. Some of the extubation parameters described in neuromuscular respiratory failure and their predictive values are shown in Table 24.1. Oropharyngeal function is hard to assess in an intubated patient, and neck flexion or shoulder shrug do not predict failure. Often the patient is extubated, seemingly doing well and holding his own, only to deteriorate with increased work of breathing, shallow breathing, and gradual rise in arterial PCO2. In our patient example, this deterioration was also further complicated by acute mucus plugging that resulted in reintubation.

Several tests have been developed that might be useful in assessing the probability of successful extubation. One recent study proposed the use of a so-called white card test. This white card is placed 1 to 2 cm from the end of the endotracheal tube and any moisture present on the card following two to three coughs is considered a positive test. The patients are positioned with the head of the bed at 30 to 45 degrees and coached to cough maximally. It is unclear whether this test is a better predictor than a simple clinical assessment of cough strength. Another possibility is to place the patient on a spontaneous breathing trial and observe respiratory frequency and tidal volume for about an hour. We recommend that, extubation can be followed by bilevel positive airway pressure (BiPAP) noninvasive ventilation, which augments airflow and maintains positive airway pressure in the inhalation and exhalation phases.

TABLE 24.1 **Predictors for Successful Extubation Parameters in Myasthenia Gravis**

| Test | Predictive Value |
| --- | --- |
| Secretion volume | Good |
| T-piece trials (with assessment of rapid shallow breathing) | Good |
| Normal chest X-ray | Good |
| Neurologic examination (oropharyngeal function, head-flexion strength) | Uncertain |
| White card test | Uncertain |
| Pulmonary function tests | Poor |

The strongest risk factor for extubation failure in myasthenic patients is the presence of atelectasis on chest X-ray. Patients may also fail extubation if there is a significant secretion volume (an arbitrary judgment), evidence of a recent yet not sufficiently treated pneumonia, and pulmonary edema prior to extubation. It should also be pointed out that the respiratory pump needs sufficient strength and thus pyridostigmine is key. It is very difficult— and probably too stressful for the patient—to try weaning the ventilator without pyridostigmine. Simply said, breathing does not work if the bellows don't work.

Finally patients may also develop post-extubation stridor. One recently noted complication is that vocal cord abduction paralysis may occur in the anti-MuSK variant of myasthenia gravis.

So after these events how should we proceed with our patient? How can we get the infected secretions under control and wean from the ventilator safely? It was decided to place a tracheostomy, and after a week, cultures came back with a multiresistant pseudomonas that was treated with aerosolized colistin. The patient gradually improved, although multiple bronchoscopies were needed to clear the secretions. A gradual decrease in pyridostigmine possibly also contributed to the decrease in secretions, and the patient was transitioned—in incremental steps—to pressure support and eventually to spontaneous breathing trials.

Treatment of myasthenia gravis with acute neuromuscular respiratory failure takes time. In our patient it took about 6 weeks before he could be dismissed from the hospital. Patients with myasthenia gravis and difficulties getting off of the ventilator often have had prior episodes of crisis, and in these cases a prolonged period of hospitalization can be anticipated.

---

**KEY POINTS TO REMEMBER REGARDING WEANING OF THE VENTILATOR IN MYASTHENIA GRAVIS**

- Reintubation is common in myasthenia gravis, especially in patients with bronchial hypersecretion and atelectasis.
- Long-term management with placement of a tracheostomy is needed after reintubation.
- Finding an optimal dose of pyridostigmine after treatment of myasthenic crisis is difficult. There is a fine line between minimizing

- secretions and optimizing the strength of oropharyngeal and respiratory muscles.
- PLEX is the preferred treatment in myasthenic patients with severe neuromuscular respiratory muscle weakness.
- PLEX may not be sufficient to wean a patient off the ventilator, and pyridostigmine is needed to improve respiratory muscle function.

**Further Reading**

Chaudhuri A, Behan PO. Myasthenic crisis. *QJM* 2009; 102:97-107.

Frutos-Vivar F, Ferguson ND, Esteban A et al. Risk factors for extubation failure in patients following a successful spontaneous breathing trial. *Chest* 2006; 130:1664-1671.

Jani-Acsadi A, Lisak RP. Myasthenia gravis. *Curr Treat Options Neurol* 2010; 12 231-243.

Khamiees M, Raju P, DeGirolamo A, Amoateng-Adjepong Y, Manthous CA. Predictors of extubation outcome in patients who have passed a trial of spontaneous breathing. *Chest* 2001; 120:1262-1270.

Lacomis D. Myasthenic crisis. *Neurocrit Care* 2005; 3:189-194.

Mandawat, A., Kaminski, H. J., Cutter, G et al. Comparative analysis of therapeutic options used for myasthenia gravis. *Ann. Neurol* 2010;68: 797-805

Mandawat A, Mandawat A, Kaminski HJ et al. Outcome of plasmapheresis in myasthenia gravis: delayed therapy is not favorable. *Muscle Nerve* 2011;43:578-584

Seneviratne J, Mandrekar J, Wijdicks EFM, Rabinstein AA. Predictors of extubation failure in myasthenic crisis. *Arch Neurol* 2008; 65:929-933.

Sylva M, van der Kooi AJ, Grolman W. Dyspnoea due to vocal fold abduction paresis in anti-MuSK myasthenia gravis. *J Neurol Neurosurg Psychiatry* 2008; 79:1083-1084.

# 25 Hyponatremia After Subarachnoid Hemorrhage

A 46-year-old woman with history of smoking and hypertension developed a thunderclap headache associated with emesis but no loss of consciousness. On arrival to the emergency department she was mildly confused and had no focal neurological deficits (World Federation of Neurological Surgeons—WFNS—Scale grade I). Head CT scan showed subarachnoid hemorrhage with aneurysmal pattern and mildly dilated ventricles. Her admission serum sodium level was 140 mmol/L. She was admitted to our neurosciences ICU, and a lumbar drain was placed, with resulting improvement of her headache and confusion. The following morning she had a cerebral angiogram, which revealed an anterior communicating artery aneurysm. The aneurysm was coiled without complications. She remained well over the following three days but developed increasing polyuria and a progressive decline in serum sodium. On day four she was still mostly asymptomatic but we noticed subtle new cognitive difficulties. We rechecked a transcranial Doppler and noticed that the mean blood flow velocities in the first segments of both anterior cerebral arteries and the right middle cerebral artery were increased by 30-40% compared with the previous day. Despite consistently receiving 150 cc per hour of 0.9% sodium chloride for the last 2 days, her fluid balance had been negative by 1.5 liters over the preceding 24 hours. Her serum sodium level has declined to 128 mmol/L from 135 mmol/L 8 hours earlier.

**What do you do now?**

Hyponatremia can occur in nearly half of cases of aneurysmal subarachnoid hemorrhage (aSAH). Serum sodium may decline at any time between 3 and 14 days after aneurysm rupture, but more commonly before the onset of cerebral vasospasm. Symptoms from hyponatremia are generally not severe. Confusion, increased drowsiness, and even seizures can occur when sodium levels are declining rapidly. Focal deficits are not caused by hyponatremia. The appearance of hyponatremia in aSAH should be considered a warning sign indicating the possibility of intravascular volume contraction, which can be particularly concerning in the setting of cerebral vasospasm.

Hyponatremia and volume contraction go hand in hand because the main cause of hyponatremia in aSAH is cerebral salt wasting syndrome. This is a disorder characterized by excessive secretion of natriuretic peptides leading to increased urinary sodium loss. In turn, the increased sodium in the urine drags water with it. The consequences are polyuria and intravascular volume depletion. Patients with aSAH may also have the syndrome of inappropriate secretion of antidiuretic hormone (SIADH), which produces excessive retention of free water at the tubular level and results in dilutional hyponatremia. The problem is that readily available tests of the blood and urine are not very useful to differentiate SIADH (associated with normal or mildly expanded intravascular volume) from cerebral salt wasting (associated with intravascular volume contraction) (Figures 25.1 and 25.2). Cerebral salt wasting typically predominates, as reflected by the frequent improvement of hyponatremia after infusion of isotonic saline in these patients (isotonic fluid administration worsens hyponatremia associated with SIADH).

Determining the volume status of the intravascular compartment in aSAH is extremely difficult and most times it can only be roughly estimated. Monitoring the central venous pressure may help, but the reliability of this measurement is limited. We, like many others, have moved away from using pulmonary artery catheters in most of these patients. Novel noninvasive methods appear promising, but they have not been sufficiently validated. Thus, since there are no ideal ways to gauge the volume status, it is most prudent to assume that polyuric patients with worsening hyponatremia will develop volume contraction.

When treating patients with aSAH we must therefore replace fluid volume and sodium. Hypertonic saline can achieve this goal. We often start

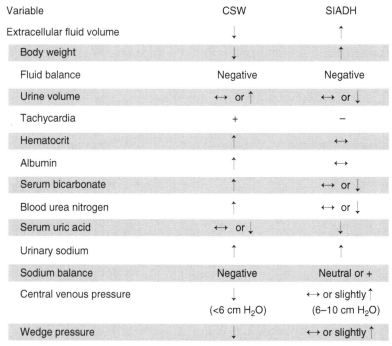

| Variable | CSW | SIADH |
|---|---|---|
| Extracellular fluid volume | ↓ | ↑ |
| Body weight | ↓ | ↑ |
| Fluid balance | Negative | Negative |
| Urine volume | ↔ or ↑ | ↔ or ↓ |
| Tachycardia | + | − |
| Hematocrit | ↑ | ↔ |
| Albumin | ↑ | ↔ |
| Serum bicarbonate | ↑ | ↔ or ↓ |
| Blood urea nitrogen | ↑ | ↔ or ↓ |
| Serum uric acid | ↔ or ↓ | ↓ |
| Urinary sodium | ↑ | ↑ |
| Sodium balance | Negative | Neutral or + |
| Central venous pressure | ↓ (<6 cm H₂O) | ↔ or slightly ↑ (6–10 cm H₂O) |
| Wedge pressure | ↓ | ↔ or slightly ↑ |

**FIGURE 25.1** Differential diagnosis between cerebral salt wasting (CSW) and syndrome of inappropriate secretion of antidiuretic hormone (SIADH).

with 1.5% sodium chloride, but resort to 3% solution if the hyponatremia is severe or fails to improve with lower concentration of sodium replacement. If hyperchloremic acidosis develops, we switch to sodium acetate, adjusting the concentration to maintain the same tonicity. Our therapeutic goal is to correct the hyponatremia and, most importantly, to maintain euvolemia.

Some patients with aSAH become extremely polyuric, and this tends to occur at the peak of cerebral vasospasm. In these situations it is all too common that we get stuck in a vicious circle of giving more crystalloid fluids to compensate for the unrelenting fluid and sodium loss. One must scale back fluid administration to avoid complications such as pulmonary edema or renal medullary washout.

Mineralocorticoids are useful to prevent or ameliorate excessive urinary excretion and hyponatremia in patients with aSAH. Only early initiation

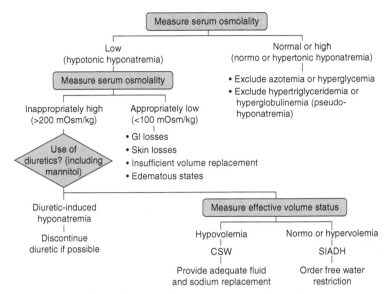

**FIGURE 25.2** Algorithm for the evaluation and management of hyponatremia in a critically ill neurological patient. CSW, cerebral salt wasting; SIADH, syndrome of inappropriate secretion of antidiuretic hormone.

(within 72 hours of aneurysm rupture) has been formally tested and proven effective. In placebo-controlled studies, fludrocortisone was associated with fewer side effects than hydrocortisone (which may cause hyperglycemia due to its glucocorticoid activity), but neither medication increased the risk of congestive heart failure. In our practice, we start fludrocortisone (0.2 mg twice daily) early in most patients with aSAH (higher doses of fludrocortisone may be needed in refractory cases).

Hypotonic intravenous fluids (Table 25.1) should be avoided in patients with aSAH, not only because hyponatremia is so frequent but also because these patients are at increased risk of intracranial hypertension. In alert patients tolerating an oral diet, the tonicity and sodium concentration of ingested fluids should also be regulated. These patients usually get thirsty as they become polyuric, and abundant ingestion of water may exacerbate the hyponatremia. In these cases, we have patients drink fluids enriched with high concentrations of sodium (attempting to treat hyponatremia with sodium tablets or salty foods is inefficient).

TABLE 25.1 **Sodium Content in Common Intravenous Fluid Solutions**

| Intravenous fluid | Sodium content (mmol per liter) |
| --- | --- |
| 5% dextrose* | 0 |
| 0.45% sodium chloride* | 77 |
| Ringer's Lactate* | 130 |
| 0.9% sodium chloride† | 154 |
| 1.5% sodium chloride† | 256 |
| 3% sodium chloride†** | 513 |

* Not recommended for use in aneurysmal subarachnoid hemorrhage
† Recommended for use in aneurysmal subarachnoid hemorrhage
** Requires central access

We treated our patient with fludrocortisone and increased volume of 1.5% sodium chloride. Her sodium level improved progressively despite persistent polyuria and it returned to normal range 48 hours later. She also developed fluctuating alertness that we attributed to diffuse cerebral vasospasm, which resolved with hemodynamic augmentation therapy (phenylephrine infusion). She was discharged home after 15 days of hospital stay and returned to work 5 weeks later.

Hyponatremia is a common concern in patients with aSAH, and its pathophysiology is not completely understood. It should be considered an indicator of volume contraction, and its treatment is hypertonic saline. Fludrocortisone can help prevent this complication. Fluid restriction may substantially increase the risk of cerebral infarction in patients with hyponatremia and cerebral vasospasm and therefore it should be avoided.

### KEY POINTS TO REMEMBER REGARDING HYPONATREMIA AFTER SUBARACHNOID HEMORRHAGE

- Hyponatremia is common after aneurysmal subarachnoid hemorrhage and it is often associated with intravascular volume contraction.
- Treatment of the polyuric, hyponatremic patient should include replacement of sodium and fluid volume.

- The goals of fluid management in cases of aneurysmal subarachnoid hemorrhage are maintenance of normonatremia and euvolemia.
- One must replace volume effectively, but being careful not to induce fluid overload.
- Fludrocortisone is useful to ameliorate urinary sodium loss and hyponatremia.

### Further Reading

Audibert G, Steinmann G, de Talancé N et al. Endocrine response after severe subarachnoid hemorrhage related to sodium and blood volume regulation. *Anesth Analg* 2009; 108:1922-1928.

Brimioulle S, Orellana-Jimenez C et al. Hyponatremia in neurological patients: cerebral salt wasting versus inappropriate antidiuretic hormone secretion. *Intensive Care Med* 2008; 34:125-131.

Hasan D, Wijdicks EF, Vermeulen M. Hyponatremia is associated with cerebral ischemia in patients with aneurysmal subarachnoid hemorrhage. *Ann Neurol* 1990; 27:106-108.

Harrigan MR. Cerebral salt wasting syndrome: a review. *Neurosurgery* 1996: 38:152-160.

Rabinstein AA, Bruder N. Management of hyponatremia and volume contraction. *Neuro Crit Care* 2011; in press.

Rabinstein AA, Wijdicks EF. Hyponatremia in critically ill neurological patients. *Neurologist* 2003; 9:290-300.

Rahman M, Friedman WA. Hyponatremia in neurosurgical patients:clinical guideline development. *Neurosurgery* 2009:65:925-935.

Sterns RH, Hix JK, Silver S. Treatment of hyponatremia. *Curr Opin Nephrol Hypertens* 2010:19:493-498.

Sterns RH, Silver SM. Cerebral salt wasting versus SIADH: what difference? *J Am Soc Nephrol* 2008; 19:194-196.

Wijdicks EF, Vermeulen M, Hijdra A, van Gijn J. Hyponatremia and cerebral infarction in patients with ruptured intracranial aneurysms: is fluid restriction harmful? *Ann Neurol* 1985; 17:137-140.

Wijdicks EF, Vermeulen M, ten Haaf JA et al. Volume depletion and natriuresis in patients with a ruptured intracranial aneurysm. *Ann Neurol* 1985; 18:211-216.

Diabetes Insipidus After Brain Tumor Surgery

A 40-year-old woman was evaluated for recurrent suprasellar pilocytic astrocytoma causing worsening headaches, visual loss, and hydrocephalus (Figure 26.1A). In the distant past her tumor had been treated with debulking and radiation. She was taking cabergoline to control her excessive prolactin production, levothyroxine for her hypothyroidism, and dexamethasone for treatment of tumor swelling. Until a couple of months ago she had been using low-dose DDAVP (desmopressin acetate) for diagnosis of central diabetes insipidus, but this medication had been discontinued after she developed hyponatremia. As a first step she underwent ventriculoperitoneal shunt placement with improvement of her symptoms. Six weeks later she was readmitted for tumor resection. The surgical approach was interhemispheric, transcallosal, and transventricular. Despite extensive adhesions to adjacent structures the tumor was successfully removed (Figure 26.1B). The pituitary infundibulum was noted to be infiltrated by the tumor. Within hours of the surgery, the patient developed marked polyuria (1.4 liters over the previous 90 minutes). Her serum sodium level has increased to 146 mmol/L from 138 mmol/L,

serum osmolality is 297 mOsm/kg, urine osmolality is
113 mOsm/kg, and urine specific gravity is 1.003.

A

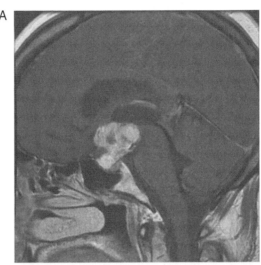

B

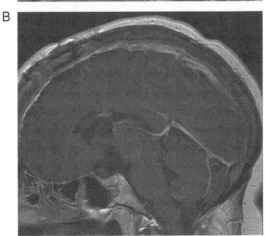

**FIGURE 26.1** A) Preoperative MRI scan showing a large suprasellar enhancing mass with
associated obstructive hydrocephalus. B) Postoperative MRI scan showing complete
resection of the previously observed suprasellar mass. (Both MR images are gadolinium-
enhanced sagittal T1 sequences.

Polyuria and hypernatremia after craniotomy point to a defect in vasopressin secretion. Neurosurgery in the region, particularly if transsphenoidal causes deficiency of arginine-vasopressin (AVP) secretion and central diabetes insipidus (DI) (Table 26.1). AVP increases the permeability to water of the renal cells lining the distal tubules and medullary collecting ducts. With AVP deficiency, water is not reabsorbed and large quantities of diluted urine are excreted. Patients can become rapidly dehydrated and develop severe hypertonic hypernatremia if their water intake is insufficient to compensate the loss. Ambulatory patients get thirsty and may maintain a balance through drinking large amounts of fluids (polydipsia).

TABLE 26.1  **Causes of Central Diabetes Insipidus in the NICU**

Brain tumors*

    Pituitary adenoma

    Craniopharyngioma

    Pilocytic astrocytoma

    Meningioma

    Hypothalamic hamartoma

    Metastasis

    Lymphoma

Transsphenoidal neurosurgery*

Brain death*

Traumatic brain injury*

Langerhans cell histiocytosis

Erdheim Chester disease (non–Langerhans cell histiocytosis)

Sarcoidosis

Wegener's granulomatosis

Subarachnoid hemorrhage

Sheehan's syndrome (postpartum ischemic pituitary necrosis)

Asterisk indicates common causes in the NICU

Critically ill and postneurosurgical patients depend entirely on the health care team to administer them enough fluids. With a severe disturbance, AVP needs to be fully replaced.

When evaluating a neurological patient with polyuria—usually defined as 24-hour urinary excretion > 50 ml/kg of body weight—the first necessary piece of information is the serum sodium concentration. If the patient is markedly hypernatremic and the hypernatremia is not iatrogenic (e.g., after large doses of hypertonic saline or mannitol), the diagnosis of DI is very likely. The diagnosis is supported if the urine is hypotonic (urine osmolality < 300 mOsm/kg, urine specific gravity < 1.010) despite hypertonic serum. Moreover, the major improvement in urine concentration that follows the administration of DDAVP confirms the diagnosis.

The management of DI is more complicated than appreciated. Physicians need to follow the changes in serum sodium concentration and fluid balance very closely. The management of hypertonic hypernatremia from DI starts by maximizing adequate water replacement. One has to administer enough fluids to prevent or correct hypovolemia. Sodium chloride 0.9% (normal saline solution) is often quite hypotonic in relation to serum sodium concentration in these patients and it is the intravenous solution we generally use first, unless the degree of hypernatremia is becoming dangerously high (> 160 mmol/L). It is important to be cautious about the administration of hypotonic intravenous solutions to patients at risk of postoperative brain swelling, and we favor a less aggressive replacement of the free water deficit in these patients than usually recommended.

Calculating the free water deficit is useful to adequately treat patients with central DI. The formula for this calculation is:

$$\text{Free water deficit} = \text{Normal TBW} - \text{Current TBW}$$

where normal TBW (total body water) is 60% of lean body weight in kilograms in men and 50% in women, and current TBW is calculated as follows:

$$\text{Current TBW} = \text{Normal TBW} \times (140/\text{current serum sodium level})$$

Once the free water deficit is known, one can calculate the amount of fluids to give depending on the fluid tonicity:

$$\text{Replacement fluid volume (in liters)} = \text{Free water deficit} \times (1/1 - X)$$

where X = replacement fluid sodium concentration – isotonic fluid sodium concentration (refer to Table 25.1 for information on sodium concentration in commonly used intravenous fluids).

As these formulas fail to tell us how the serum sodium concentration will change as we replace the fluid, we have found the following alternative formula to be useful in practice:

$$\text{Change in serum Na} = \text{replacement fluid Na} - \text{serum Na/normal TBW} + 1$$

This formula tells us how much the serum sodium concentration will change after the retention of 1 liter of the replacement fluid.

It is prudent to avoid rapid swings in serum sodium concentration. The risk of myelinolysis is unknown when correcting hypernatremia compared to hyponatremia, but we still prefer to reduce hypernatremia by not more than 10 mmol/L per day. In addition, and most important, patients with postoperative brain swelling could potentially worsen if a high serum sodium level is corrected too quickly. In such patients, lowering the sodium but maintaining a more moderate degree of hypernatremia may be a better therapeutic target.

Oral intake and enteral administration (via gastric tube) of free water are safe. We have seen patients in whom small volumes of intravenous hypotonic fluids were detrimental while large volumes of free water given by nasogastric tube were not. As a consequence, we prefer gastric free water flushes for the gradual correction of hypernatremia in neurocritical patients.

We start DDAVP when the polyuria is severe (more than 500 mL per hour for two consecutive hours or an average of more than 300 mL per hour over 4 hours) and when the serum sodium concentration is rising fast. We may start with a low dose, such as 1 microgram intravenously. Typically the urinary output begins to slow down within 15–20 minutes. If the response is insufficient after 60 minutes, we repeat a higher dose (1–2 micrograms). Monitoring of urinary output and serial serum sodium measurements should guide the timing of the next dose. Because gastric absorption may be poor in these patients, we prefer intravenous administration until we can be confident that we have defined a daily requirement and the situation is stable. At that point we may switch to nasal (or oral) formulations. Chlorpropamide (sometimes combined with a thiazide) has also been used to treat central DI. Although it is indeed a potent antidiuretic, we rarely administer this medication because it can provoke severe hypoglycemia.

Patients with aneurysmal subarachnoid hemorrhage who develop central DI represent another challenge. DI is relatively uncommon, but it may present early after rupture of a midline aneurysm and mostly in patients who present with poor clinical grade. The onset is sudden, and the hypernatremia can be quite severe, but the duration is short and it is generally followed by cerebral salt wasting. DDAVP and hypotonic intravenous fluids need to be used very cautiously in these patients as they may contribute to the abrupt occurrence of severe hyponatremia. This shift from hypernatremia to hyponatremia can also occur in patients with traumatic brain injury, but the change is slower. Finally, diabetes insipidus may be one of the first signs that a patient is meeting criteria for brain death. Usually hypotension accompanies the development of polyuria and hypernatremia (chapter 31).

Our patient was treated with a combination of crystalloids (a combination of 0.9% and 0.45% sodium chloride), enteral free water, and DDAVP (first intravenously and then orally after several days). Her stay in the ICU was extended by a week as a result of the need to closely monitor her labile DI. Eventually she recovered well except for short-term memory deficits

### TABLE 26.2  Protocol to Treat Diabetes Insipidus

STABLE HYPERNATREMIA (<150 mmol/L)

Monitor polyuria and match with fluid intake

Consider free water (250 ml) flushes through NG tube

Monitor body weight, urine specific gravity

RISING OR SEVERE HYPERNATREMIA

Start desmopressin 1 mcg IV and repeat if inadequate response (max 4 mcg/d in divided doses)

Start 0.45% sodium chloride or 5% dextrose and calculate infusion rate (see text)

Monitor serum sodium every 2–4 hours.

Monitor urine specific gravity

likely due to fornix injury. Six months later, her urinary production and serum sodium levels were stable on oral DDAVP (0.4 mg twice daily). As it was the case in our patient, it is not uncommon that patients with brain tumors, brain trauma, or after neurosurgery need long-term treatment with DDAVP. These patients need a comprehensive endocrine evaluation for possible panhypopituitarism. In fact, even in the absence of signs of pituitary apoplexy, investigation of adrenal and thyroid function should be considered in any patient with central DI in the ICU.

A protocol to treat diabetes insipidus is shown in Table 26.2.

### KEY POINTS TO REMEMBER REGARDING DIABETES INSIPIDUS AFTER BRAIN TUMOR SURGERY

- Postoperative polyuria after surgery for a suprasellar tumor should promptly raise suspicion of diabetes insipidus.
- Diabetes insipidus can be a component of panhypopituitarism in patients with brain tumor, brain trauma, and infiltrating granulomatous diseases.
- Diabetes insipidus in a catastrophically injured patient may be one of the first signs of brain death.
- Diagnosis of diabetes insipidus is based on the presence of polyuria associated with hypernatremia, serum hyperosmolality, and urine hypoosmolality.
- Management of central diabetes insipidus consists of aggressive rehydration and intravenous administration of DDAVP.
- Be wary of giving hypotonic intravenous fluids to patients with brain swelling. Lowering serum sodium to a more moderate degree of hypernatremia primarily by administering free water through the gastric tube is a safer strategy in these patients.

**Further Reading**

Adrogue HJ, Madias NE. Hypernatremia. *N Engl J Med* 2000; 342:1493-1499.

Jane JA, Vance ML, Laws ER Neurogenic diabetes insipidus *Pituitary*. 2006; 9:327-329.

Krahulik D, Zapletalova J, Frysak Z, Vaverka M. Dysfunction of hypothalamic-hypophysial axis after traumatic brain injury in adults. *J Neurosurg* 2010; 113:581-584.

Kristof RA, Rother M, Neuloh G, Klingmüller D. Incidence, clinical manifestations, and course of water and electrolyte metabolism disturbances following transsphenoidal pituitary adenoma surgery: a prospective observational study. *J Neurosurg* 2009; 111:555-562.

Nemergut EC, Dumont AS, Barry UT, Laws ER. Perioperative management of patients undergoing transsphenoidal pituitary surgery. *Anesth Analg* 2005; 101:1170-1781.

Rabinstein AA, Wijdicks EFM. Body water and electrolytes. In: *Textbook of Neurointensive Care.* (Layton AJ, Gabrielli A, Friedman WA eds), 2004, pp 555-577, Saunders, Philadelphia.

Verbalis JG. Management of disorders of water metabolism in patients with pituitary tumors. *Pituitary* 2002:5:119-132.

A 71-year-old female with a prior history of a glioblastoma, treated with radiation and temozolomide, was admitted with new-onset, generalized, tonic-clonic seizures. The patient had developed a recent deep venous thrombosis that required warfarin. Because she failed to maintain an adequately opened airway she was emergently intubated and—because of an allergy to phenytoin—she was treated with intravenous levetiracetam before transfer to the neurological intensive care unit. After admission, the patient received an additional dose of 2 grams of IV levetiracetam because of recurrent seizures, and after another seizure she also received valproic acid (1100 mg as a loading dose followed by 500 mg IV b.i.d.). Seizures were adequately controlled with this combination. The next day, the international normalized ratio (INR), which was measured basically as a routine follow-up, is 5.5 (increased from admission INR of 3.0), and a repeat INR hours later was 7.6. Brain MRI scan shows a glioma with large amount of vasogenic edema, but no evidence of a recent hemorrhage. Intratumoral blood products could be seen in the gradient recalled echo (GRE) sequence.

## What do you do now?

It has been known for years that a single memorable experience with a drug interaction is needed to make physicians aware of that interaction. Without such experience—usually leading to a potential complication—physicians are not typically aware of major drug interactions and certainly not the less frequent ones. Fortunately, most of the drug interactions are clinically inconsequential and do not require adjustments.

Drug interactions are expected in critically ill patients—as a result of polypharmacy. Drug interactions can lead to medical complications, and best known are QTc prolongation, hypokalemia, hypotension, hypertension, and cardiac arrhythmias.

Drug interactions in a neurosciences intensive care unit (NICU) are often different from those caused by commonly used drugs in medical and surgical intensive care units. Although theoretically there are many, the 5 most common interactions in NICU are shown in Table 27.1. Any physician rotating through or attending in the NICU should be cognizant of these interactions, but in our experience they are often unrecognized. ICU pharmacists have been helpful in identifying these drug interactions early and in pointing out their pharmacokinetic basis.

One class of drugs that are mostly used in NICU are antiepileptic drugs, and that is where the unfamiliarity among physicians is the greatest. One such significant effect is that most antiepileptic drugs increase metabolism of warfarin and therefore *decrease* its effect. This has important repercussions if these antiepileptic drugs are suddenly discontinued, which could lead to sudden increase in warfarin effect. The only antiepileptic agent that increases the action of warfarin and therefore causes a significant *increase* in INR is valproic acid. Both drugs—warfarin and valproic acid—are acidic compounds with a small volume of distribution and they are highly protein bound. There is a high affinity for the same binding site on human albumin. Therefore, competition for albumin-binding sites between these drugs results in displacement of warfarin from albumin-binding sites and a transient increase in INR. In anticoagulated patients, displacement of less than 1% of total plasma warfarin can result in significant change of warfarin action.

Our patient is a typical example of such an interaction. This drug interaction is more profound if valproic acid is given in a large (loading) dose, and thus anticoagulated patients receiving a loading dose of valproic acid should have their INR closely monitored. INR may rise substantially and

TABLE 27.1  **The 5 Drug Interactions You Need to Know About in the NICU**

Warfarin and Valproic acid

*Mode of action*: Drug displacement in protein binding site; a high loading dose reaching a higher serum level may displace warfarin from of valproic acid binding site.

Phenytoin and Fluconazole

*Mode of action*: Fluconazole inhibits phenytoin metabolism and may increase phenytoin level up to 4 times. Serum concentration monitoring with a reduction in phenytoin dosage is warranted.

Valproic acid and Carbapenems

*Mode of action*: The exact mechanism is unknown. Carbapenems, especially meropenem, may inhibit valproic acid absorption. Meropenem may accelerate the renal excretion and may result in low valproic acid serum level and increase risk of seizures. Additionally, carbapenems lower seizure threshold.

Statin and Levofloxacin or Amiodarone

*Mode of action:* The exact mechanism is unknown, but severe rhabdomyolysis may occur.

Clopidogrel and Omeprazole

*Mode of action:* Omeprazole inhibits CYP2C19, which is responsible for the conversion of clopidogrel into its active form. The effect of clopidogrel is reduced up to 47%.

may potentially lead to bleeding either spontaneously or in areas prone to bleed (e.g., tracheostomy sites, prior wound beds, recent ischemic or hemorrhagic stroke, recent craniotomy, recent brain biopsy or ventriculostomy.) Our patient received 10 mg of vitamin K and fresh frozen plasma and did not develop any bleeding complication.

In situations where acute decisions will have to be made—such as with our patient—drug interactions may not be on the radar, but it is important to consider the effects antiepileptic drugs have on anticoagulation. The antiepileptic drug that seems to have the safest profile is levetiracetam. Most importantly the frequent use of antiepileptic drugs in the NICU requires knowledge of their effects on other drugs and on other antiepileptics. These are summarized in Table 27.2.

TABLE 27.2 **Drug Interactions with Antiepileptic Drugs**

| | |
|---|---|
| | *Decreases effect* |
| Phenytoin | Theophylline |
| | Corticosteroids |
| | (dexamethasone) |
| | Warfarin |
| Carbamazepine | Phenytoin |
| | Warfarin |
| Barbiturates | Phenytoin |
| | Corticosteroids |
| | Tricyclic |
| | antidepressants |
| | Warfarin |
| | *Increases effect* |
| Valproic acid | Warfarin |

### KEY POINTS TO REMEMBER REGARDING DRUG INTERACTIONS

- Most antiepileptic drugs decrease INR, and valproate increases INR, in patients receiving warfarin.
- Sudden discontinuation of antiepileptic drugs can result in marked increase in INR and lead to bleeding complications.
- Many antiepileptic drugs decrease the effect of commonly used drugs including corticosteroids and tricyclic antidepressants.

**Further Reading**

Bertsche T, Pfaff J, Schiller P, et al. Prevention of adverse drug reactions in intensive care patients by personal intervention based on an electronic clinical decision support system. *Intensive Care Med* 2010; 36:655–672.

Guthrie SK, Stoysich AM, Bader G, Hilleman DE. Hypothesized interaction between valproic acid and warfarin. *J Clin Psychopharm* 1995; 15:138–139.

Juurlink DN, Mamdani M, Kopp A, Laupacis A, Redelmeier DA. Drug-drug interactions among elderly patients hospitalized for drug toxicity. *JAMA* 2003; 289:1652-1658.

Ko Y, Malone DC, D'Agostino JV, Skrepnek GH, Armstrong EP, Brown M, Woosley RL. Potential determinants of prescribers' drug-drug interaction knowledge. *Research in Social and Administrative Pharmacy* 2008; 4:355-366.

Moura C, Prado N, Acurcio F. Potential drug-drug interactions associated with prolonged stays in the intensive care unit: a retrospective study. *Clin Drug Investig* 2011;31:309-316.

Reimche L, Forster AJ, van Walraven C. Incidence and contributors to potential drug-drug interactions in hospitalized patients. *J Clin Pharmacol* 2011; 51:1043-1050.

Seller EM, Koch-Weser J. Kinetics and clinical importance of displacement of warfarin from albumin by acidic drugs. *Annals of the New York Academy of Sciences* 1971; 179:213-225.

# Long-term Support, End-of-Life Care, and Palliation

# 28 Decisions in Persistent Vegetative State

A 17-year-old teenager remained comatose 2 weeks after a severe traumatic brain injury. During the first days following the accident, he was treated for refractory increased intracranial pressure associated with multiple frontal and temporal lobe contusions. A frontal decompressive craniectomy was needed at some point. His clinical course was complicated by seizures, pulmonary infection, and bacteriemia. Early decubital redness appeared. After resolution of the intracranial hypertension no change in his neurologic examination was noted, and he has stayed comatose. He has not developed sleep and wake cycles. On examination, he has his eyes open at times, but is not tracking a finger, nor fixating on his parents when they are in the room. A loud handclap does not produce any reaction. He grinds his teeth. There is spontaneous extensor posturing. He may sweat profusely occasionally.

All clinical indicators point toward the development of a persistent vegetative state. The nursing staff has not noticed any signs of awareness, but the family is not so sure. Long-term support is desired. There are questions by the family members whether improvement can occur and at what level the patient might be able to function.

**What do you do now?**

Outcome prediction in young patients after severe traumatic brain injury is a necessary task for neurosurgeons and neurologists. When patients display clinical signs of a persistent vegetative state and also have neuroimaging documentation of severe brain injury, the need for long-term care will come up and decisions will have to be made.

There are multiple prediction models in head injury. The largest database of traumatic head injury (IMPACT; International Mission for Prognosis and Analysis of Clinical trials in Traumatic brain injury) uses admission characteristics to calculate a prognosis estimate. These are age, motor response, pupil responses, presence of hypoxia and hypotension, CT categorization into severity of lesions and presence of a mass lesion, presence of traumatic subarachnoid hemorrhage, epidural mass, and also serum glucose and hemoglobin values (calculator at www.tbi-impact.org). In our patient example, the predicted 6 months mortality is 64% and predicted 6 months unfavorable outcome (death, vegetative state, and severe disability) is 83%. Hopeful parents will be encouraged by these numbers. Physicians will express serious doubt. Every physician involved with long-term care of traumatic brain injury will know that we can never be certain and prediction in young comatose patients with intact brainstem reflexes has serious limitations.

The general guide is that if the clinical findings of persistent vegetative state are still present after 3 months in nontraumatic coma (i.e., anoxic-ischemic encephalopathy, hypoglycemia, CNS infections, status epilepticus) substantial recovery of awareness is not anticipated. In traumatic brain injury, 12 months are needed for reasonable certainty, but recovery to a minimally conscious state may occur beyond this time limit.

There has been renewed interest in persistent vegetative state and the accuracy of the clinical diagnosis. The diagnosis of persistent vegetative state is well defined (Table 28.1). The common questions have been: Is persistent vegetative state truly persistent? Is our neurologic examination reliable? Do we have better ways to assess "consciousness?" Can functional MRI scans predict recovery? Can functional MRI scans find evidence of some awareness not detected clinically? The reliability of neurological examination has withstood the test of time, although errors by non-neurologists are still considerable. Some of the above questions cannot be answered yet with certainty.

TABLE 28.1  **Clinical Signs of Persistent Vegetative State**

Breathing regular (with tracheostomy in place)

Bronchial hypersecretion

Blood pressure stable

Immobile

Flexion-extension contractures

Eyes closed or open

No evidence of focus or holding attention

No eye movements to examiner (except briefly when suddenly confronting)

Eyes roving, nystagmoid, gaze preference changing, no eye contact for more than 5 seconds

Eyes may move upward or downward or assume lateral gaze for 1-2 minutes

No sound (if not made impossible with tracheostomy)

Spontaneous teeth grinding

Spontaneous clonus, or shivering

Functional MRI scan remains a research tool, but brain activation on a functional MRI does not mean consciousness.

Once long-term care has been decided, a tracheostomy and percutaneous endoscopic gastrostomy (PEG) should be placed, often simultaneously (Table 28.2). Common contraindications for a PEG are: active coagulopathy, inability to perform endoscopy (pharyngeal obstruction), prior abdominal surgery involving the stomach, and most importantly, uncertainty about need for long-term care (it is poor medical practice to place a tracheostomy and PEG if care is withdrawn weeks later).

Usually a general surgeon will perform these procedures. Enteral feeding is discontinued 12 hours before surgery. Antibiotic prophylaxis to reduce peristomal infection is administered, and feeding can be started 24 hours or less after placement. Complications are quite infrequent and some can be anticipated. Pneumoperitoneum is common due to air escaping through the stomach opening and is only concerning when peritonitis occurs.

**TABLE 28.2 Precautionary Measures with Gastrostomy and Tracheostomy**

Checks with gastrostomy placement

INR < 1.5; platelets > 50,000/mm³
Discontinue intravenous heparin or antiplatelet agents (5 days)
Cefotaxime 2 gram IV single dose
Fasting for 4-6 hours
Anticipate use of midazolam (may need airway protection)
Resume tube feeding 1 hour after placement
Monitor for pneumoperitoneum with upright chest X-ray
Monitor white blood cell counts with fever

Checks with tracheostomy placement

BMI < 30 kg/m²
Stable cervical spine fracture
No high PEEP (< 10 cm $H_2O$) or high FiO2 requirements
INR < 1.5; platelets > 50,000/mm³
Discontinue intravenous heparin
Anticipate oxygen desaturation
Anticipate hypotension
Anticipate bleeding at site

BMI: Body Mass index; PEEP: positive end expiratory pressure; FiO2: fraction of inspired oxygen; INR: international normalized ratio.

Air can be obscured by concomitant pulmonary infiltrates, and upright X-ray of the chest is needed to make the diagnosis in these cases.

The advantages of tracheostomy in permanently comatose patients are substantial. These include ease of suctioning, reduced requirement of sedation, shorter duration of mechanical ventilation and ability to transfer patients to a long-term facility. Timing of tracheostomy placement has been a topic of debate. Early performance of tracheostomy (sometimes as early as within the first week of mechanical ventilation) has been proposed in patients expected to require prolonged mechanical ventilation; however, the value of this practice has not been proven. We favor the more conservative approach of proceeding with a percutaneous tracheostomy at least 10 days after the start of mechanical ventilation and when need for more than 3 weeks of mechanical ventilation is anticipated. Direct tracheostomy (i.e., without previous endotracheal intubation) may be needed in severe neck and facial trauma or when there is inability to secure an airway. Complications of percutaneous tracheostomy are very uncommon when done by skilled surgeons (less than 2%), but percutaneous tracheostomy cannot be considered in patients with possible cervical neck injury, morbid obesity, and significant coagulopathy. Continuous need for intravenous heparin may make management of the bleeding site also difficult. Eventually patients will have the tracheostomy down-sized. Uncomplicated plugging of the tube for several days ("corking") indicates that decannulation can be considered.

Long-term care in a nursing home facility is needed, and patients are typically followed by physicians who face a continuous challenge to prevent and treat infections. Superb nursing care and physical therapy are essential to prevent early and late fatal complications.

---

**KEY POINTS TO REMEMBER REGARDING DECISIONS IN PERSISTENT VEGETATIVE STATE**

- Prognostication after traumatic head injury can be assisted by the use of large database models (such as IMPACT), but these models are far from perfect.
- Persistent vegetative state is considered permanent one year after traumatic brain injury, but already permanent 3 months after nontraumatic coma. There are exceptions.
- Tracheostomy and PEG are essentially part of the decision to maintain best long-term support of the patient and should be considered early.

**Further Reading**

Bernat JL. Chronic disorders of consciousness. *Lancet* 2006; 367:1181-1192.

Durbin CG. Tracheostomy: why, when, and how? *Respir Care* 2010; 55:1056-1068.

Lingsma HF, Roozenbeek B, Steyerberg EW, Murray GD, Maas AI. Early prognosis in traumatic brain injury: from prophecies to predictions. *Lancet Neurol* 2010; 9:543-554.

Kornblith LZ, Burlew CC, Moore EE et al One thousand bedside percutaneous tracheostomies in the surgical intensive care unit: Time to change the gold standard. *J Am Coll Surg* 2011;21:163-170.

Koc D, Gercek A, Gencosmanoglu R et al. Percutaneous endoscopic gastrostomy in the neurosurgical intensive care unit: complications and outcome. *JPEN J Parenter Enteral Nutr* 2007;31:517-520.

Loser C, Aschl G, Hebuterne X, Mathus-Vliegen EMH, Muscaritoli M, Niv Y, Rollins H, Singer P, Skelly RH. ESPEN guidelines on artificial enteral nutrition–percutaneous endoscopic gastrostomy (PEG). *Clinical Nutrition* 2005; 24:848-861.

Wijdicks EFM. The Comatose Patient. Oxford University Press, New York, 2008.

Do-Not-Resuscitate Orders and Withdrawal of Life Support

A 78-year-old woman is admitted to the NICU with a destructive ICH (large ganglionic hemorrhage involving the diencephalon, Figure 29.1) On examination, she has midsize fixed pupils but with preserved corneal reflexes and a good cough response and she overbreathes the ventilator. She has flexion withdrawal of both arms with nail bed compression in the fingers and triple flexion responses of the legs.

The family arrives and wants "everything done." The family is very clear about her: She is a fighter and in the past was able to overcome desperate situations in which physicians had given up any hope for recovery. She has told the family "do not let me go so easily." Recently, an ICD has been placed, and the family interpretation of that procedure is that this also shows she wanted to live. Therefore the family specifically requests to give her all the time she needs to recover and to resuscitate her if that were needed. The patient's condition is unchanged 3 days later.

**What do you do now?**

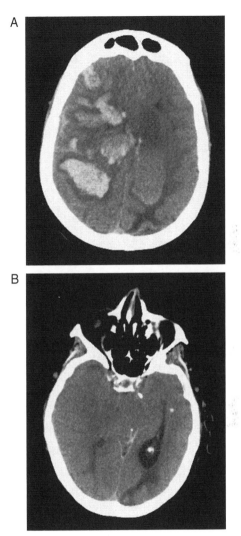

**FIGURE 29.1** CT scan showing a massive right intraparenchymal hematoma with intraventricular extension, hydrocephalus (A), and brain tissue displacement causing complete effacement of the basilar cisterns (B).

End-of-life care in the intensive care has become a shared decision-making process in the United States and such an approach is considered more satisfactory than decisions based on physician's authority alone. When asked in surveys, most families appreciate a physician's openness and directness. Families would want to know what to expect and what are the limitations of aggressive interventions. In patients with very poor prognosis it is important to review the chances of a successful resuscitation effort.

Where did a do-not-resuscitate (DNR) order originate? In 1974, the American Medical Association stated in an article devoted to standards that "cardiorespiratory resuscitation was not indicated in certain situations." Other opinions were voiced, including the 1983 President's Commission on "deciding to forego life sustaining support." This led to a major change in practice, in which doctors now had the opportunity to discuss any intervention before the event. Most major medical organizations supported the view that do-not-resuscitate orders can be discussed as part of care. How to communicate this to family members or even whether to discuss the actual procedure of cardiopulmonary resuscitation has remained an underdeveloped field of medicine, and training of this part of end-of-life care in residencies is generally not common place.

What do the data say about the success of cardiopulmonary resuscitation in the intensive care unit? In most large series of resuscitated critically ill patients with diverse diagnoses not more than 15% survive to discharge. Advanced age and comorbidity (i.e., cancer) reduce the odds even more. Patients with acute deteriorating neurologic disease complicated by cardiac arrest and cardiopulmonary resuscitation have a very dismal outcome, if they survive at all. Some empirical guidelines in patients with acute neurologic disease are clearly warranted, but none exist. In an earlier statement there appeared to be consensus among stroke physicians that DNR orders are appropriate if 2 of the 3 following criteria are met: 1) severe deficit, persistent or deteriorating and with impaired consciousness; 2) life-threatening brain damage with brainstem compression involving multiple brainstem levels; 3) significant comorbidity, including pneumonia, pulmonary emboli, sepsis, recent myocardial infarction, and life-threatening arrhythmias. Criteria for other critical neurologic conditions have not been developed, but most physicians attending in the NICU would discuss DNR orders—if not already made clear by family members—or an advance directive, if there is permanent and severe primary brain and brainstem injury.

A DNR order clearly specifies no cardiopulmonary resuscitation (no chest compressions, no pharmacologic or electrical cardioversion). Do not intubate orders (no endotracheal intubation or invasive mechanical ventilation) typically accompany the DNR order, but exceptions occur. Orders limiting aggressive care may also prohibit use of noninvasive (BiPAP) mechanical ventilation, intravenous drugs or infusions for cardiac arrhythmias with preserved circulation, cardiac pacemakers, or chest tubes, among other supportive devices indicative of aggressive care. However, it is important to keep in mind that a DNR order per se should not affect the level of care provided to the patient except obviously in the case of a cardiac arrest. Other restrictions of medical treatment or de-escalation of care should be specified separately from the DNR order.

These distinctions are crucial to avoid unintended problems with a DNR order. Some studies have found that DNR orders may negatively influence triage to the ICU. Some patients may feel that DNR order may impact aggressiveness of care. Multiple studies have found that certain cultures will see a DNR order as equivalent to withholding treatment. It should not. In some situations DNR could be the first step toward de-escalation of care. However, in itself DNR merely defines the limits of care.

In the United States surrogates are able to make decisions, and they could be guided by advance directives. A living will directs proxy to withhold or withdraw treatment at the end of life. A living will is usually formulated in broad terms (often containing a sentence such as, "if I have terminal disease I do not want to be resuscitated"), and obviously rarely includes specifics on acute neurologic disease. Decision makers for the patients therefore will have to interpret such a will. Nonetheless the mere fact a living will exists indicates that the patient has anticipated that a difficult medical situation may occur in the future. It expresses a wish by the patient to assist family members in making such decisions.

So what should we do in this situation? Providing factual information is the first course of action, and this requires a formal family conference (Table 29.1). Sitting down and having a conversation in a separate room is far more appropriate than a cursory discussion at the bedside. Physicians may need to use visual aids (showing the large destructive hemorrhage),

**TABLE 29.1  The Family Conference (10 Steps)**

1. Sit down in a quiet place (separate room)

2. Identify yourself

3. Summarize recent developments

4. Proceed with a summary of the clinical course

5. Summarize the big picture and treatment goals

6. Estimate and describe disability

7. Discuss tracheostomy and gastrostomy

8. Discuss palliative care

9. Discuss code status

10. Answer questions

establish trust under stressful circumstances, and may need multiple conversations which should include having the family summarize the assessment of the situation. Physician should respect cultural and religious beliefs, but these may be an impediment to rational medical care. In many families considerable time may be needed to grasp the finality of the condition.

Explanations should relay specific information (Table 29.2). If the patient has worsened, the family should understand why the patient has worsened. In some situations a third party may be helpful in the discussions, and a medical ethics committee may be able to resolve differences if

**TABLE 29.2  Information to Convey to Family Members When Discussing Do-Not-Resuscitate**

| | |
|---|---|
| Procedure: | Chest compression, defibrillation, intubation, mechanical ventilation, invasive catheters, medications; may mean 20–30 minutes with poor brain perfusion |
| Outcome: | 2/3 survive resuscitation; 1/10 survive to discharge |
| Consequences: | Care otherwise not different<br>Cardioversion still option if needed<br>Aggressive ICU care continues (e.g., hemodialysis still optional) |

there is an emerging conflict between the patient's family and the treating physician. In fact, withholding or withdrawing treatment is a common reason for consulting the medical ethics committee. Ethics consultants may be able to spend additional time with the family—lack of time is often a limiting factor in the communications in the ICU—explaining the issues at hand with equanimity and compassion. Yet, it remains to be seen whether ethics committees can defuse conflict once a very antagonistic family–physician relationship has developed.

How did we approach this quandary? The family in this particular patient example was told that it was very likely she was going to remain comatose and cardiopulmonary resuscitation could bring her heartbeat back, but she would not be able to recover important function needed to understand her situation. After daily conversations with the family about the patient's condition, it became clear all of them understood the gravity of the brain injury. In these discussions long-term care using a tracheostomy and gastrostomy was brought up. The family eventually decided that long-term care was not in her best interest and a do-not-resuscitate order was placed. Several days later the family decided to withdraw the ventilator and to provide palliative care only.

The case illustrated here represents an extreme in the spectrum of severity of acute brain damage, but it is a common clinical scenario in NICUs. It was clear to all of us upon arrival that she could not recover, even with the most aggressive supportive treatment. Yet, several family conferences were necessary before the family accepted that their loved one would not regain consciousness. By the time they requested that life support measures be withdrawn, they were at peace with their decision and appreciative of the time we had spent with them and the care the patient had received.

Families expect an estimate of outcome. What we say as neurologists about prognosis and the way we deliver this message may greatly influence decisions on subsequent level of care. This responsibility must be accepted with full understanding of its weight.

When communicating a poor prognosis leads to limitations in the level of care or withdrawal of life support, a *self-fulfilling prophecy* may occur. This philosophy has received considerable attention in the literature over the last decade. Some have even provocatively claimed that the prognosis of a poor outcome might be the single factor most strongly associated with mortality in patients with intracerebral hemorrhage. Our prognostic abilities are imperfect, and we should be aware of this possibility. We should also be mindful of exaggerations or trivialization in the discussion of this important topic.

The *point of no return*, a condition incompatible with survival or meaningful recovery, is expected with severe brainstem injury, but defining the boundary of good, not too bad, and poor outcome has proven far more difficult than it seems. Useful indicators of poor prognosis—often loss of pontomesencephalic reflexes and coma—have been described, but almost invariably the studies supporting their predictive value have not accounted for the potential influence of withdrawal of life support or restriction of aggressive care measures. In other words, an intracerebral hematoma volume exceeding 60 cc has been consistently associated with high mortality and poor recovery, but death in these patients is often preceded by withdrawal of life support, and prognostic studies have rarely accounted for this caveat or provided more neurologic detail. Finding a solution to this limitation of studies on prognosis is very difficult because it would require analyzing a population of patients treated aggressively even after clinicians feel that such care has become frankly futile. It also would require very detailed analysis of the neurological condition. For example, a comatose patient with a destructive hemorrhage and persistent loss of several brainstem reflexes and extensor posturing is not expected to improve substantially, but a patient with spared brainstem reflexes might, and in such cases withdrawal of life support may be sometimes too premature.

The other important issue to keep in mind is that cognitive and physical incapacity rather than death is the outcome most feared by the great majority of patients and families. The key question we are asked by families is not whether the patient can survive the acute brain insult but whether survival can be followed by meaningful functional recovery (admittedly the word "meaningful" in this setting carries a certain arbitrariness). Studies evaluating the possible occurrence of the self-fulfilling prophecy using mortality as the main endpoint fail to address this point. In addition, even the most detailed statistical analysis may be insufficient to account for the effect of the combination of catastrophic brain disease and previous chronic illnesses in an elderly and previously debilitated patient. In all honesty we may not have the answer in all medical conditions, but it would be concerning—and create for physicians a truly unworkable environment—if the concept of self-fulfilling prophesy were to become a pretext to keep patients alive at whatever effort and cost.

Withdrawal of life support measures consists of extubation and discontinuation of any administered drugs. Central access and arterial catheters are removed, and the monitor is turned off. In our institution, we may start a morphine infusion of 0.1 mg/kg/hr and titrate to comfort by increasing infusion with small increments every 15 min until the patient is "comfortable." We may institute a lorazepam infusion of 0.05 mg/kg/hr and titrate upward slowly until symptoms of agitation or restlessness are controlled. In deeply comatose patients none of this is indicated unless breathing after extubation becomes markedly labored. Most patients with brainstem injury die within hours after life support is withdrawn. Transfer to a palliative care room—in the event the patient remains stable—is desirable.

---

**KEY POINTS TO REMEMBER REGARDING DO-NOT-RESUSCITATE ORDERS AND WITHDRAWAL OF LIFE SUPPORT**

- Do-not-resuscitate orders may be warranted in catastrophic neurologic injuries.
- The appropriateness of cardiopulmonary resuscitation (full code) depends on the probability of good outcome and absence of life-shortening comorbidity.
- Repeated conversations with family members are extremely important, and time should be reserved to do so in an appropriate way.
- End of life care should include discussions with surrogates using a shared decision model.
- Decisions should include a broad picture of validated predictors of outcome, previous functional status, coexistent illnesses and patient's preferences.
- Difficult situations may be resolved with the assistance from a hospital ethical committee.

## Further Reading

Alexandrov AV, Pullicino PM, Meslin EM, Norris JW. Agreement on disease-specific criteria for do-not-resuscitate orders in acute stroke. Members of the Canadian and Western New York Stroke Consortiums. *Stroke* 1996; 27:232-237.

Becker KJ, Baxter AB, Cohen WA et al. Withdrawal of support in intracerebral hemorrhage may lead to self-fulfilling prophecies. *Neurology* 2001; 56:766-772.

Bernat JL. Ethical aspects of determining and communicating prognosis in critical care. *Neurocrit Care* 2004; 1:107-117.

Burns JP, Edwards J, Johnson J et al. Do-not-resuscitate order after 25 years. *Crit Care Med* 2003; 31:1543-1550.

Curtis JR, Tonelli MR Shared Decision-making in the ICU. *Am J Respir Crit Care Med* 2011;183:840-841.

Rabinstein AA. Ethical dilemmas in the neurologic ICU: withdrawing life-support measures after devastating brain injury. *Continuum* 2009; 15:13-25.

Rabinstein AA, McClelland RL, Wijdicks EFM et al. Cardiopulmonary resuscitation in critically ill neurologic-neurosurgical patients. *Mayo Clin Proc* 2004; 79:1391-1395.

Tian J, Kaufman DA, Zarich S et al. Outcomes of critically ill patients who received cardiopulmonary resuscitation. *Am J Resp Crit Care Med* 2010; 182:501-506.

White DB, Braddock CH III, Bereknyei S, Curtis JR. Toward shared decision making at the end of life in intensive care units: opportunities for improvement. *Arch Intern Med* 2007; 167:461-467.

Wijdicks EFN, Rabinstein AA. Absolutely no hope? Some ambiguity of futility of care in devastating acute stroke. *Crit Care Med* 2004; 32:2332-2342.

Wijdicks EFN, Rabinstein AA. The family conference: end-of-life guidelines at work for comatose patients. *Neurology* 2007; 68:1092-1094.

# Pitfalls of Brain Death Determination

A 20-year-old graduate student, sideswiped while driving at an intersection, was found comatose by paramedics. He was emergently intubated and admitted to the surgical trauma unit. He had multiple frontal and temporal lobe contusions, a pelvic fracture, and pulmonary contusions. He had no motor response to pain, pupils were fixed and dilated, and he did not grimace to pain. He lost his pulse and required cardiopulmonary resuscitation for 30 minutes.

Neurosurgery placed an intracranial pressure monitor that showed initial normal (< 20 mm Hg) intracranial pressure (ICP) readings, but ICP later increased to 40-50 mmHg, not responding to osmotic diuretics. Blood pressures remained unstable, requiring vasopressors. The trauma surgeon believes the patient is brain dead, as the patient stopped triggering the ventilator. You are asked to do a formal brain death examination. Upon questioning, the intensive care nurse tells you that the patient is not on any sedative drugs and fentanyl infusion was discontinued 4 hours ago.

**What do you do now?**

Severe traumatic brain injury may result in admission to a neurosciences intensive care unit (NICU) or a surgical trauma intensive care unit when there are additional multiple injuries. In most parts of the world neurosurgeons and neurologists determine whether the patient meets the clinical criteria of brain death. These patients may be in a designated NICU, but they can also be in other ICUs. Not being the attending physician means you need more time to understand the time course of events and interventions that have taken place. Commonly the situation and request for the determination of brain death are not crystal clear.

Any physician making the clinical diagnosis of brain death should work through a predetermined set of criteria. It starts with the recognition of "red flags," confounders which neurologists recognize as unacceptable and which generally, when present, should make everyone uncomfortable to even proceed to a more formal neurological examination (Table 30.1). More difficult is the opposite situation. There may be an unnecessary delay of brain death determination, if certain clinical findings are misinterpreted as not compatible with the diagnosis of brain death (Table 30.2).

The question that is most often asked is: How long should one wait until a patient can be declared brain dead? The answer—of course—is as long as it takes to determine a treatment is futile and to exclude possible confounders. Patients admitted to ICUs who have deteriorated from a major brain injury may "look" imminently agonal, but aggressive treatment—in some— could lead to substantial improvement. It is therefore premature to declare

---

TABLE 30.1 **Signs that the Patient May Not Be Brain-Dead**

Insufficient time of observation (any transfer from an outside hospital is
potentially suspect for presence of sedative or neuromuscular blocking drugs)

Cause of coma not established

Treatable cause of coma

Fever and shock

Hypothermia (< 32° C)

Unsupported blood pressures, no need for vasopressors

Evidence of substantial alcohol or drug intake

TABLE 30.2  **Signs Compatible with Brain Death**

Spinal cord reflexes (neck-arm flexion, arm lifting, head turning, triple flexion response)

Ventilator, not patient, auto-triggering (ventilator at fault and auto-triggering due to minor changes in pressure or volume in the circuit)

Intracranial blood flow preserved

Presence of some EEG activity

---

a patient's brain death with an active CNS infection, untreated brain edema, undrained hydrocephalus, non-decompressed mass effect, any major uncorrected laboratory abnormality, or marked hypothermia. In these patients some previously absent brainstem reflexes and motor responses can return. However, when all brainstem reflexes are lost in a demonstrable apneic patient and there is no other explanation these findings are irreversible.

Excluding sedative drugs does require calculation of time to elimination (the sum of 5 half-lives is conservative). The most common drugs are fentanyl (t ½ = 6 hours), lorazepam (t ½ = 15 hours), midazolam (t ½ = 6 hours), phenobarbital (t ½ = 100 hours), and thiopental (t ½ = 20 hours). If patients have been treated with therapeutic hypothermia or if there has been ischemic liver injury after cardiopulmonary resuscitation, it will be very difficult—if not actually impossible—to exclude a lingering sedative effect. Most neuromuscular junction blockers are eliminated within several hours (the commonly used atracurium t ½ = 30 minutes), but the simplest proof of its lack of effect is the return of tendon reflexes. Bedside nerve stimulators can also be used. Other potentially complicating medical conditions are hypothermia (usually less than 32°C), severe hyponatremia (< 110 mmol/L), hypernatremia (> 160 mmol/L), hypoglycemia (< 40 mg/dL), or hypercalcemia (>3.4 mmol/L).

The actual neurologic evaluation of determining brain death consists of 25 tests and verifications. Brain death determination is complex (it is more than checking a few brainstem reflexes in an apneic patient), requires expertise (hopefully a neurologist or neurointensivist), and demands perfect diagnostic accuracy (no room for error). The overriding principle is simple: establish cause, determine futility, exclude confounders, examine brainstem reflexes, and test for apnea. Many physicians have difficulty with the apnea test, but the test—a $CO_2$ challenge using oxygen-diffusion—is simple and safe when its steps are carefully followed (The procedure is described in Table 30.3).

One examination suffices in adults, but some U.S. states require 2 physicians to examine the patient. In infants and children (30 days to 18 years), repeat examinations are recommended: 2 examinations by 2 separate examiners, and 12 hours apart. In neonates (newborn with at least 37 gestational weeks to 30 days), 2 examinations by 2 separate examiners, but 24 hours apart are required (these new recommendations are based on a consensus report sponsored by the Society of Critical Care Medicine and American Academy of Pediatrics). The clinical examination always concludes with an apnea test, and the time of completion of this test is the time of death. A checklist is shown in Table 30.3.

Confirmatory tests (or better called ancillary tests) may have far less specificity than previously appreciated. These tests may not fit the clinical examination. In fact, retained blood flow is just a reflection of the intracranial pressure, which may not be high enough to stop blood entry through the dura into the skull (in other words, very high ICP: no flow; high but not very high ICP: retained flow). The same applies to electrodiagnostic tests; they are just a reflection of cortical function and not brainstem function. To use these tests to shorten observation time or to declare brain death— assuming no flow or no electrical brain activity—in patients with confounding drug effects or even intoxication will only lead to errors. No physician wants to declare a patient brain-dead using a confirmatory test to override a confounder and be told by the nursing staff that there has been return of motor movement or spontaneous breathing. Nonetheless, these ancillary tests are mandatory in some countries in Europe, Latin America, and Asia. Sometimes it seems that the focus in brain death determination has unfortunately shifted to finding an ideal technical test rather than improving clinical competence.

So what should you do? The patient likely suffered anoxic-ischemic injury in addition to traumatic diffuse axonal and contusional brain injury, and reversal of this condition is not likely. In this patient it is prudent to wait another day (5 half-lives of fentanyl is 30 hours – 4 hours of discontinuation = 26 hours). A drug screen should be obtained to exclude drugs the patient may have co-ingested (alcohol level, serum toxicological screen).

TABLE 30.3 **Twenty-Five Assessments to Declare a Patient Brain-Dead**

**Prerequisites** (all must be checked)

1. Coma, irreversible and cause known
2. Neuroimaging explains coma
3. CNS depressant drug effect absent
    (*if indicated, order toxicology screen; if barbiturates given, serum level < 10 mcg/ml*)
4. No evidence of residual paralytics
    (*Peripheral nerve stimulator, if paralytics used*)
5. Absence of severe acid-base, electrolyte, endocrine abnormality
6. Normal or near normal temperature
    (*Core temperature ≥ 36°C*)
7. Systolic BP ≥ 100 mmHg
8. No spontaneous respirations

**Examination** (all must be checked)

9. Pupils nonreactive to bright light
10. Corneal reflexes absent
11. Eyes immobile, oculocephalic reflex absent
    (*tested only if C-spine integrity ensured*)
12. Oculovestibular reflex absent
13. No facial movement to noxious stimuli at supraorbital nerve, TMJ; (*absent snout or rooting reflexes in neonates*)
14. Gag reflex absent
15. Cough reflex absent to tracheal suctioning
16. Absence of motor response to noxious stimuli in all 4 limbs (*Spinally mediated reflexes are permissible, and triple flexion reflex is most common*)

**Apnea Testing** (all must be checked)

17. Patient is hemodynamically stable (*BP > 90 mm Hg*)
18. Ventilator adjusted to provide normocarbia
    (*$PaCO_2$ 35-45 mmHg*)
19. Patient preoxygenated with 100% $FiO_2$ for >10 minutes to $PaO_2$ > 200 mmHg
20. Patient maintains oxygenation with a PEEP of 5 cm of water
21. Disconnect ventilator

(*Continues*)

TABLE 30.3 **(Cont'd.)**

| | |
|---|---|
| 22. | Provide oxygen via an insufflation catheter to the level of the carina at 6 liters/min or attach T-piece with CPAP valve at 10 cm $H_2O$ |
| 23. | Spontaneous respirations absent |
| 24. | ABG drawn at 8–10 minutes, patient reconnected to ventilator |
| 25. | $PCO_2 \geq 60$ mmHg, or 20 mmHg rise from normal baseline value, document time of death |
| | or |
| | Apnea test aborted and ancillary test (EEG or blood flow study) confirmatory, document time of death |

Adapted from Wijdicks et al., 2010.
ABG = arterial blood gas; BP = blood pressure; CPAP = continuous positive airway pressure; PEEP = positive end expiratory pressure; TMJ = temporomandibular joints

Brain death determination allows closure and options for organ donation. There is no medical rationale to continue care if there is no consent for organ donation. No intensive care unit has the obligation to care for a legally deceased person, and in the extreme it would be unethical if holding the bed can cause refusal of necessary transfers of other patients.

> **KEY POINTS TO REMEMBER REGARDING BRAIN DEATH DETERMINATION**
>
> - Brain death determination is time-consuming and involves multiple tests.
> - Most time should be spent in finding possible confounding factors.
> - The diagnosis is based on a clinical neurologic examination and not on cerebral blood flow or an electrodiagnostic study.
> - Two examinations by 2 separate physicians are needed in infants and children.
> - In the U.S. one examination is sufficient in adults (> 18 years).
> - Some U.S. states require 2 physicians to examine the patient usually at approximately the same time.
> - Confirmatory tests are legally necessary in some countries

**Further Reading**

Jain S, DeGeorgia JS. Brain death-associated reflexes and automatisms. *Neurocrit Care* 2005; 3:122-126.

Lustbader D, O'Hara D, Wijdicks EF, MacLean L, Tajik W, Ying A, Berg E, Goldstein M. Second brain death examination may negatively affect organ donation. *Neurology*. 2011;76:119-124.

Nakagawa TA, Ashwal S, Mathur M, Mysore M, and the Committee for Determination of Brain Death in Infants and Children. Guidelines for the determination of brain death in infants and children: an update of the 1987 task force recommendations *Crit Care Med* 2011, in press.

Wijdicks EFM, Varelas PN, Gronseth GS, Greer DM et al. Evidence-based guideline update: determining brain death in adults: report of the Quality Standards Subcommittee of the American Academy of Neurology. *Neurology* 2010; 74:1911-1918.

Wijdicks EFM. The case against confirmatory tests for determining brain death in adults. *Neurology* 2010; 75:77-83.

Wijdicks EFM. There is no reversible  braindeath. *Crit Care Med* 2011; 39:2204-2205.

A 51-year-old man with poorly controlled hypertension and severe congestive heart failure was admitted with a devastating ganglionic hemorrhage. Soon after arrival he was intubated in the emergency department. About 2 hours after the onset of signs the patient had his eyes closed with no opening to temporomandibular pressure, fixed midsize pupils, absent corneal reflexes, minimal oculovestibular responses, but a good cough response after tracheal suctioning. He also had spontaneous extensor posturing and triple flexion responses with Babinski signs. The CT scan showed a large destructive ganglionic hemorrhage starting in the putamen and extending into the frontal lobe and diencephalon. There was trapping of the third ventricle and acute hydrocephalus. In a desperate and likely ineffective attempt to improve the neurologic condition, a ventriculostomy was placed, but the consulted neurosurgeon felt there was no benefit in removing the large hematoma with so many brainstem reflexes lost. Over the next hours more brainstem reflexes disappeared, and only a faint cough reflex and a breathing drive remained, as evidenced by triggering of the ventilator.

The family understood very well that there was no chance to salvage him and they were told that he might progress further and become brain-dead within several hours. The family brought up his previously expressed strong desire for organ donation if something major would happen to him. However, 24 hours after admission to the neurological intensive care unit, the neurologic examination has remained unchanged. The family would still like to donate his organs after withdrawal of support.

*What do you do now?*

Catastrophic neurologic injury is often quite obvious even within hours after presentation. In such extreme cases, acute neurosurgical intervention or other measures to reduce increased intracranial pressure are futile. In these acute circumstances with rapid onset of coma, neurologists and neurosurgeons try to identify "a point of no return," and that is mostly defined by the degree of destruction, by the involvement of crucial structures maintaining awareness (i.e., the diencephalon), and by persistent upper brainstem dysfunction. Clinically this translates into no pupillary light responses, no corneal responses, and no oculocephalic responses. The lower part of the brainstem (lower pons and medulla oblongata) is often still functioning, as made clear by the presence of a motor response to a noxious stimulus, a cough response to tracheal suctioning, and the patients' preserved ability to trigger a ventilator.

In these situations when there is no hope for recovery, withdrawal of intensive care support will rapidly come up during a family conference, and often the decision is to provide palliative care after extubation.

It is easy to see that something good may come out of such a deep distress, and we should agree with the family, that if feasible, organ donation should be explored. Two clinical scenarios are expected. First, a considerable proportion of these patients will eventually progress to loss of all brainstem function and can be officially declared brain-dead and be therefore legally deceased. Organ donation can then be discussed, and the procedures are well established. But, if the patient does not meet the clinical criteria for brain death, the patient could potentially become a candidate for donation after withdrawal of life support. This procedure is known as donation after cardiac death protocol (abbreviated "DCD protocol"). It requires two important decisions: to establish with certainty the presence of a hopeless situation and when to withdraw life-support measures. Proponents of a DCD protocol have claimed a significant increase in donation rates, but the increase has still been less conspicuous than hoped for.

A DCD procurement protocol is more complicated and restricted than a brain death procurement protocol. Important differences between the two protocols are shown in Table 31.1.

Many hospitals in the United States—in order to maintain accreditation—are now required to have a DCD protocol in place; however, few physicians are fully aware of their responsibilities within these protocols. The utilization

TABLE 31.1 **Differences between a Donation after Cardiac Death (DCD) and Donation after Brain Death (DBD) Protocols**

| Variables | DCD | DBD |
| --- | --- | --- |
| Preconditions | No confounders and irremediable cause | No confounders and irremediable cause |
| Clinical findings | Devastating neurologic injury and often loss of upper brainstem function. | Coma, absent brainstem reflexes, no motor response and apnea |
| Eligibility Determination | Preferably an independent physician | Attending physician (may need confirmation by another physician) |
| Organ recovery | 5 minutes circulatory arrest after patient extubation in the operating room | Immediately after arrival |
| Organ/tissue | All those consented except heart (lungs rarely procured) | All those consented |
| Triage | May return to ICU for palliative care if patient breathes after extubation | Morgue |

of DCD protocols worldwide is more variable, with marked differences in utilization between Asian and European countries. Most notable is the absence of DCD protocols in Germany.

In brief, the DCD protocol is based on organ retrieval after circulatory arrest. After withdrawal of life support has been decided, the patient may become a candidate for a DCD protocol. The eligibility is decided by an organ procurement coordinator and it requires a detailed conversation with the family, a signed informed consent, a determination of organ suitability, and a match with a recipient. A detailed medical and social history is obtained from the family. Contraindications to organ donation may include infectious diseases (notably HIV and hepatitis C), potentially transmissible malignancies (possibly including primary brain tumors manipulated by biopsy or ventriculostomy), and, most commonly, unsuitable organs. Blood (or tissue) samples are sent to a laboratory designated by the organ procurement organization for serological testing and tissue typing. The family should be made aware that the entire DCD procedure may take about 24 to 36 hours to complete. During this time the patient is examined regularly because progression to brain death may still occur. This transition is dependent on the time from the injury, but such progression is not common if no neurologic deterioration has been observed for 2 days. The family should also be made aware that the patient goes still intubated to an operating room. Extubation takes place in the operating room, but after extubation the patient may breathe, and the heart may not stop. If circulatory arrest does not happen within a predefined time interval (up to 60 minutes) the DCD procedure is aborted, and the patient may have to return to the intensive care unit and later the ward for further palliative care.

So what can be expected if the family decides to go ahead? After all appropriate preparations, the patient is transferred to the operating room and prepared for organ retrieval. In the operating bed, the patient is fully draped with the thorax and abdomen sterilized. Instruments are prepared and placed on a tray. Coming to the operating room for family members is a major event and a new and likely a difficult experience. (We had nurses that had a visceral response after witnessing such a procedure and prefer not to go there anymore.) In the dimly lit serene operating room the family would sit close to the patients' head behind a sterile drape. Usually only the attending physician, an anesthesiologist, and an operating nurse and the organ procurement coordinator are present. The surgical team is out of the operating room and out of sight.

The patient is extubated. After the patient is extubated the patient will often gasp for several minutes, becoming deeply cyanotic until breathing stops. It may take several minutes for a circulatory arrest to occur (asystole is not a criterion although both often go together). The determination of circulatory arrest involves palpating the carotid artery, next to appearance of a zero reading of the invasive arterial pressure tracing. At that very moment the family is told the patient has died and is escorted out the operating room. After circulatory arrest is determined and documented, a 5-minute "death watch" begins with monitoring for any change. After 5 minutes have passed, the surgical team enters the operating room and proceeds quickly with a large splitting thoracoabdominal incision followed by rapid cooling, emptying large buckets of ice in the abdominal cavity, cannulation of major arteries, and infusion of preservation fluids and mobilization of transplantable organs. The transplant surgeon may determine on inspection that certain organs are unsuitable for organ donation. The deceased patient then goes to the morgue.

However, organ harvesting cannot take place if respiratory and circulatory arrest do not occur within one hour of extubation. In such cases, the patient is transported back to the ICU or to a regular room to receive palliative measures. These failed DCD attempts are not only costly but also can be distressing to families and discouraging to the medical team.

Respiratory and circulatory arrest in the operating room after extubation has been very difficult to predict, and most studies show about a 50/50 chance of respiratory/circulatory arrest within the 60-minute allotted observation time. Available predictive scores are not adapted for neurological patients. In one study of critically ill neurological patients the combination of absent corneal reflex, absent cough reflex, and extensor or absent motor responses predicted respiratory/circulatory arrest within 60 minutes of extubation in 85% of cases. When combined with an abnormal oxygenation index (> 4.2) the prediction increased to 93%. (Each factor alone predicted respiratory-circulatory arrest about two thirds of the time.)

The organ procurement coordinator often also will try to do a "mini apnea test" in the ICU, which is basically placing the patient on a CPAP of 5 cm of $H_2O$ and watching for respiratory deterioration. With no evidence of respiratory deterioration, the chance that the patient will develop a respiratory arrest after extubation in operating room later is smaller, and some organ procurement officers will call the procedure off and have the patient not go to the operating room. Clearly, more accurate predictors for cardiac arrest are necessary in patients with a catastrophic neurologic injury when life support is withdrawn.

DCD protocols create an important opportunity to donate tissue and organs, but the decisions—starting with the determination to withdraw support—are far more complicated and ethically challenging than in cases of donation after brain death. With an expected increase in DCD donors—still about 20% of all donors—physicians should be aware of the procedures.

**Further Reading**

Bernat JL, Capron AM, Bleck TP et al. The circulatory-respiratory determination of death in organ donation. *Crit Care Med* 2010; 38:963-670.

Dominguez-Gil G, Haase-Kromwijk B,Van Leiden H et al. Current situation of donation after circulatory death in European countries. *Transplant Int.* 2011 April 19, Ahead of print.

Frontera JA. How I manage the adult potential organ donor: donation after cardiac death (part 2). *Neurocrit Care* 2010; 12:111-116.

Frontera JA, Kalb T. How I manage the adult potential organ donor: donation after neurological death (part 1). *Neurocrit Care* 2010; 12:103-110.

Fugate JE, Rabinstein AA, Wijdicks EFM. Variability in DCD protocols: a national survey. *Transplantation* 2011; 91:386-389.

Reich DJ, Mulligan DC, Abt PL et al. ASTS recommended practice guidelines for controlled donation after cardiac death organ procurement and transplantation. *Am.J Transplant* 2009;9: 2004-2011.

Wijdicks EFM. Brain Death (2ed) Oxford University Press, New York, 2011.

Yee AH, Rabinstein AA, Thapa P, Mandrekar J, Wijdicks EFM. Factors influencing time to death after withdrawal of life support in neurocritical patients. *Neurology* 2010; 74:1380-1385.

# Index

Note: Page numbers followed by "*f*" or "*t*" refer to figures or tables, respectively.

Made in the USA
San Bernardino, CA
05 March 2013